EMPLOYEE RETENTION

Solving the Healthcare Crisis

EMPLOYEE

RETENTION

Solving the Healthcare Crisis

Rita E. Numerof

Michael N. Abrams

Health Administration Press

ACHE Management Series

Your board, staff, or clients may also benefit from this book's insight. For more information on quantity discounts, contact the Health Administration Press Marketing Manager at (312) 424–9470.

This publication is intended to provide accurate and authoritative information in regard to the subject matter covered. It is sold, or otherwise provided, with the understanding that the publisher is not engaged in rendering professional services. If professional advice or other expert assistance is required, the services of a competent professional should be sought.

07   06   05   04   03   5   4   3   2   1

Library of Congress Cataloging-in-Publication Data

Numerof, Rita E.
    Employee retention: solving the healthcare crisis / Rita E. Numerof, Michael N. Abrams.
        p. cm.
    ISBN 1-56793-197-9 (alk. paper)
    1. Medical personnel—Recruiting.   2. Employee retention.   3. Medical care—Personnel management.   I. Abrams, Michael N.   II. Title.

    R690.N86 2003
    610'.68'3—dc21

                                                                            2002038847

The paper used in this publication meets the minimum requirements of American National Standard for Information Sciences—Permanence of Paper for Printed Library Materials, ANSI Z39.48–1984. ™

Project manager: Jane Williams; Book/Cover designer: Matt Avery; Acquisition editor: Marcy McKay

Health Administration Press
A division of the Foundation of the
    American College of Healthcare Executives
1 North Franklin Street, Suite 1700
Chicago, IL 60606–3491
(312) 424–2800

*To the employees of healthcare delivery systems
whose personal dedication to making a positive difference
in other peoples' lives is among this country's greatest assets.*

Contents

Acknowledgments

WE WOULD LIKE to acknowledge the input of many of our clients, whose passion to improve the effectiveness of their organizations has become our common bond. In particular, we would like to thank Barb Smith at Miami Valley Hospital, Dr. Sue Fitzsimons at Yale-New Haven Hospital, and many others who over the years have worked with Numerof & Associates, Inc. to address the complex problems that healthcare providers face. We would also like to express our appreciation to all of the executives from hospitals and non-healthcare organizations who participated in the survey and follow-up interviews and agreed to share their insights and experience.

We would like to thank the staff of Numerof & Associates, Inc. (NAI) who challenged and forced us to clarify our ideas. In particular, we thank Gayle Shank, business analyst/consultant at NAI, for providing us with outstanding research support and content drafts that were enormously valuable in expanding the applicability of our observations. As with all such complex projects, our support staff—led by Carla Bruns, NAI's operations manager—did a wonderful job of keeping us organized and staying on top of the task of creating the written word. Our thanks also to Marcy

McKay, our editor at Health Administration Press. Her editorial skills helped to ensure that our models and explanations are accessible to all those who need to understand them.

Finally, we would like to acknowledge the sincere efforts of so many employees and managers in the healthcare industry whom we have come to know in 20 years of consulting. Their highest priority is to help patients when they are most vulnerable. We hope that the advice we offer in the following pages will do the same for them.

Introduction

EVERY SITUATION ANALYSIS evolves from an experiential context—the "data" that serve as the basis for identified trends, issues, and recommendations. This book is no exception. With over 20 years of experience consulting to healthcare organizations, the authors—partners in the strategic management consulting firm of Numerof & Associates, Inc. (NAI)—have worked through a greater variety of challenges than most hospital administrators have (thankfully) encountered in their careers.

Our projects have involved us in strategy development and implementation, merger and acquisition integration, employee retention "turnarounds," process redesign, and proactive use of employee survey data to effect cultural change and address management and employee issues before they become problems. In the course of our work, we have had the opportunity to interview countless hospital staff and managers, attend focus groups and town hall meetings, and work with clients to make sense of employee survey data and open-ended comments that employees submitted in a survey context. One thing that has always been apparent to us from our involvement with people in healthcare is that the overwhelming majority of them, managers and nonmanagers alike, are in the industry because they genuinely want to help others. Like all of us, they want to be successful in their vocation and want to feel that they are making a difference. Yet larger forces have negatively affected their working lives, frustrating, angering, and driving many of them out of the industry.

The increasing frequency with which our projects were related to the growing dissatisfaction of healthcare employees led us to do a preliminary study to learn how leading hospitals across the country perceived the employee-retention problem and what they were doing about it. What respondents told us about employee turnover was interesting. What was even more informative, however, was what was missing in their responses, even those from the most effective hospitals in the country.

We learned from the study that employee retention was still a reluctantly acknowledged problem for some of these hospitals. When it was acknowledged, it was often treated as a "cost of doing business." Even when retention was acknowledged as a problem that required action, the treatment was typically first aid—tactical fixes, some of which had definite but short-term impact. Clearly missing from the survey data and follow-up interviews was a systemic understanding of the problem. Our study confirmed for us that healthcare managers can fall victim to the same pitfalls as managers in other industries do such as complacency, "fighting the last war," and assuming that some business problems are just facts that "come with the territory." However, these problems require active intervention with strategic solutions and the recognition that turnover is merely a symptom of greater organizational issues.

Many managers in healthcare either experienced the labor shortages of the 1980s or acquired some sense of history about those times. Those shortages passed with only modest pain, as supply rose to meet demand and a more steady state soon ensued. Many such managers are complacently waiting for history to repeat itself, for things to "get back to normal." *That is not likely.*

The sources of our current problems in healthcare are multifaceted. They are an interweaving of changing baby boom demographics; societal change that opened new doors to women; economic pressures to contain spiraling healthcare costs; and well intentioned, if not always effective, efforts to apply lessons learned from production environments to the healthcare business.

At the level of our hospitals, the impact of these changes has been both complex and, to the outsider, subtle. But not to hospital employees. The work environment in many healthcare institutions has deteriorated, which is reflected in their satisfaction data as well as their turnover rates. Although our preliminary study revealed some tactics that offer some short-term relief, nothing short of a systemic approach will meaningfully solve the employee-retention problem. Such an approach must include six integrated practices or "pillars" that will dramatically change the work environment: (1) ensure role clarity; (2) establish optimal structures and accountability; (3) establish core process excellence; (4) ensure real-time availability of appropriate equipment, supplies, and tools; (5) create a patient-centered environment; and (6) design multiple patient care delivery models.

The reality is that the quality of experience available to employees in the healthcare environment must be competitive in all aspects with the employment alternatives available. In today's labor environment, with demographics driving the increased demand for healthcare that outstrips supply and abundant alternative employment options, competitiveness becomes more difficult to achieve. A new perspective on the problem is needed, one that reflects the true complexity of the issues involved and can offer insight into what must be done to make progress, including cross-industry solutions that work.

Given the central thesis of this book—that the recruitment and retention problems we face today are, in large part, the result of the massive dismantling of the infrastructure and the wholesale elimination of management roles—it is only fitting that rebuilding an appropriate infrastructure for tomorrow's healthcare organization must start with the pivotal role of the patient care manager. By systematically redefining the strategic priorities of this role and addressing the requirements to fulfill the role (such as competencies, support systems, staff, management interfaces, etc.), an organization can begin to shift the functioning of the entire enterprise. Building infrastructure to create a desirable work experience supports patient care and effectively promotes employee retention.

What we have attempted to provide in this book is a realistic prescription for addressing the root cause of retention problems in healthcare today.

Rita E. Numerof, Ph.D.
Michael N. Abrams, M.A.

CHAPTER 1

Industry Trends and Their Implications

HEALTHCARE IS OVERWHELMINGLY a people business. Its product, delivered by people, is the most personal one imaginable. The introduction of additional technology offers the promise of making the industry more efficient, but the industry's reliance on personal contact will not be substantially changed in the foreseeable future. Against this background the problem of employee turnover in the healthcare industry looms large. It is a problem that requires more in-depth understanding if it's to be resolved.

As healthcare executives intimately know, there is a human resource crisis in healthcare today. Shortages of workers throughout the industry escalated during the 1990s and will continue to grow well into the foreseeable future. The high turnover rates seen in this industry only exacerbate the problem of a declining labor pool. To combat this crisis, the mandate for healthcare executives is to introduce creative recruitment strategies, increase retention rates, and contain turnover to manageable levels. Failure at these efforts will threaten the availability and quality of healthcare services in the United States.

In this chapter we discuss the scope of the healthcare worker shortage and highlight factors underlying current trends. These trends include changes in demographics, market conditions, and healthcare financing and the dynamics of organizational culture.

HEALTHCARE PROFESSION TRENDS

Several interrelated trends have converged to amplify the problem of turnover in healthcare organizations today. A summary of these trends is presented in Table 1.1. Each profession's trends reveal implications for all involved and provide insights that can lead to preventive action.

Table 1.1: Trends That Influence the Healthcare Labor Shortage

Supply:
- Low unemployment rates for nurses
- Low enrollments in training programs for nurses
- Increasing turnover rates for healthcare workers
- Availability of alternative employment choices (settings and careers) for healthcare workers
- Lengthened educational component for pharmacist training, resulting in smaller number of new graduates
- Decreasing number of applications to pharmacy programs
- Aging workforce
- Salary disparities in hospitals for pharmacists and nurses
- Impact of payer pressures and low infrastructure investment

Demand:
- Technological advances require more occupational therapists, physical therapists, and respiratory therapists
- Increasing role of pharmacists
- Aging population, which requires more services and medications and presents more medically complex cases
- Growing importance of patient satisfaction

Table 1.2: Unemployment Rate for Registered Nurses

1989	1990	1991	1992	1993	1994	1995	1996	1997	1998	1999	2000
1.3%	1.1%	1.2%	1.1%	1.3%	1.5%	1.5%	1.4%	1.5%	1.3%	1.1%	1.0%

Source: U.S. Congressional Research Service. 2001. "CRS Report for Congress. A Shortage of Registered Nurses: Is It On the Horizon or Already Here?" Washington, DC: Government Printing Office.

Nursing

Of the 2.2 million registered nurses (RNs) employed in the nursing profession in March of 2000, 59 percent worked in hospital settings, a decline from 1988 when 68 percent of RNs worked in hospitals (U.S. General Accounting Office 2001). To make matters worse, 11 percent of nursing positions were open and unfilled at hospitals in 2000. According to the American Hospital Association, in 2001 there were 126,000 job openings for nurses at hospitals across the country, and 75 percent of all hospital personnel vacancies were for nurses (AHA 2001). In addition, the American Hospital Association reported that 75 percent of hospitals experienced difficulties recruiting nurses in 2000. As shown in Table 1.2, the unemployment rate for nurses in 2000 was at its lowest level in more than 12 years. This rate continues to remain below the unemployment rate for all healthcare professionals. Because the national unemployment rate for RNs was 1 percent in 2000, down from 1.5 percent in 1997, it's not surprising that vacancy rates are high for this group. The critical question is why.

One of the underlying trends in the nursing shortage is the dwindling supply of nursing candidates, as evidenced by decline in enrollment in bachelor's of science in nursing (BSN) programs. Enrollments have been decreasing steadily over a five-year period. As Figure 1.1 shows, between 1996 and 2000, enrollment declined

Figure 1.1: Five-Year Enrollment Trends in BSN Programs, 1996–2000

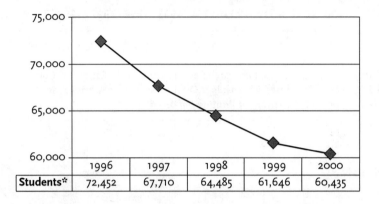

	1996	1997	1998	1999	2000
Students*	72,452	67,710	64,485	61,646	60,435

*Average decrease of 3,004 students per year

Source: Adapted with permission from American Association of Colleges of Nursing. 2000. "2000–2001 Enrollment and Graduations in Baccalaureate and Graduate Programs in Nursing." Washington, DC: AACN.

by over 12,000 students nationwide, an average decrease of 5 percent per year. Enrollment fell again in 2000 by an additional 2 percent. This downward trend is exacerbated by declining graduations from BSN programs, which fell by 23.9 percent from 1996 to 2000. Enrollment decline was also experienced in the latter half of the 1980s when the last wave of job shortages hit the healthcare industry.

To further highlight the trend, enrollments of RNs in baccalaureate programs declined by 10.4 percent from the fall of 1999 to the fall of 2000 (American Association of Colleges of Nursing 2000). This downward trend also reflects enrollment experience in masters-level nursing programs, which experienced a 4.3 percent decrease during the five-year period of 1996 to 2000. From 1999 to 2000, there was a decrease of 1.1 percent in enrollment in master's programs, which is perhaps a slight moderation of the decline (see Figure 1.2). At the same time, there is a growing demand for nurses

Figure 1.2: Five-Year Enrollment Trends in Nursing Master's Degree Programs, 1996–2000

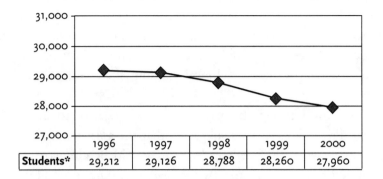

	1996	1997	1998	1999	2000
Students*	29,212	29,126	28,788	28,260	27,960

*Average decrease of 313 students per year

Source: Adapted with permission from American Association of Colleges of Nursing. 2000. "2000–2001 Enrollment and Graduations in Baccalaureate and Graduate Programs in Nursing." Washington, DC: AACN.

with advanced education to provide care to higher acuity patients, to assume nurse practitioner positions, and to prepare clinicians for a wide array of medical specialties. Those with advanced degrees also have more latitude to move into positions outside hospital settings or outside healthcare altogether, which adds to the shortage of potential candidates available to fill hospital vacancies. These three educational trends paint a bleak picture.

These factors place greater strain on the available supply of nurses to fulfill increasingly challenging clinical demands. What accounts for such dramatic declines in enrollment? Part of the answer is that more career options are available to women, who have been and continue to be the predominant enrollees of the profession. Although the BSN degree, recommended by the American Nursing Association as the base practice degree since the late 1960s, enables nurses to move beyond entry-level nursing and its corresponding compensation, this area of study is no longer as attractive as it once was. Today, the nursing profession competes with an increasing number of career choices for women, such as law, medicine, mathematics, economics, and engineering.

Declining interest in nursing careers accounts for part of the decrease in enrollments. Another consideration is the limited capacity of nursing schools to accept new enrollments because of faculty shortages, lack of clinical training sites, and insufficient classroom space.

Just how big a problem is the decline relative to projected needs? Predictions in 1988 suggested that the anticipated demand for nurses with BSN degrees by 2005 would be almost twice as great as the available supply. By the year 2015, 114,000 jobs for full-time equivalent RNs are expected to go unfilled nationwide (U.S. Department of Health and Human Services 1996). This gap will widen over the next five to ten years. A study published in the *Journal of the American Medical Association* predicts there will be a shortage of more than 400,000 RNs nationwide in 2020; this number constitutes 20 percent of the demand (Buerhaus, Auerbach, and Staiger 2000).

Adding to the supply problem is the problem of retention. The Bureau of National Affairs (2001) estimated that in 2000 turnover in healthcare as a whole—20.4 percent—was almost five percentage points higher than the average turnover in other industries, which was 15.6 percent. During the first half of 2001, overall turnover in healthcare did decrease to 18 percent and the comparable figure for other industries was 14.4 percent, reflecting a general overall tightening of the job market as a result of the softening economy. However, other surveys indicated that turnover rates for overall hospital nursing staff rose to 26.2 percent in 2000 (Hospital & Healthcare Compensation Service 2001). Sharp increases were also seen in nursing homes and home health care agencies, which had reported nursing turnover rates of 21 percent to 51 percent during the same period. What this suggests is that although overall healthcare turnover rates may be declining parallel with the economy, nursing-specific turnover is increasing at an alarming rate.

Table 1.3: ACT Scores of Healthcare Program Applicants

Program	1997	1998	1999	2000	2001	Change
Nursing (Practical)	16.8	16.8	17.0	17.0	17.0	Slight increase
Nursing (Registered)	18.6	18.6	18.6	18.6	18.6	No change
Occupational Therapy/ Assistant	19.9	19.9	19.8	19.8	19.6	Slight decrease
Pharmacy	21.7	21.6	21.5	21.3	21.2	Steady decrease
Physical Therapy/ Assistant	20.5	20.4	20.3	20.2	20.0	Steady decrease
Respiratory Therapy/Tech	17.8	17.9	18.0	18.2	17.9	Steady increase then drop

Source: Data from ACT. 1997–2001. "National Reports; Distribution of Planned Educational Majors and ACT Composite Scores." [Online information]. www.act.org.

Clearly, these trends constitute a growing crisis. Declining enrollments in bachelor's and master's degree programs, coupled with high turnover rates for healthcare and other employment opportunities, have and will continue to lead to critical shortages of nurses throughout the industry.

The educational caliber of individuals who enter nursing programs has not changed significantly over the last few years. As Table 1.3 indicates, from 1997 to 2001 ACT (college entrance exam) scores had actually increased slightly for those interested in practical nursing and had held steady for RN applicants. Note that these scores decreased for applicants to occupational therapy, pharmacy, and physical therapy programs.

Pharmacy

Are the trends described above unique to the nursing profession or are they broader? Unfortunately, there are similar trends for pharmacists in the present and future environment. The role of the pharmacist has expanded in healthcare. Pharmacists today provide a broader range of services than was true ten years ago. This is especially apparent in hospitals, where pharmacists participate in multidisciplinary clinical care teams that treat medically complex cases. In addition, medications have become increasingly complex, requiring more counseling for patients on their proper use, more drug monitoring, and more education for staff to ensure safe administration. The continued introduction of new drugs requires ongoing education for pharmacists, enabling them to update and provide their knowledge to other members of clinical care teams as well as to patients. These factors have elevated the responsibilities of the pharmacist and increased the demand for their services. How has the supply kept up and how well are hospitals, in particular, doing in attracting these essential staff members?

In 2000, approximately 30 percent of pharmacists were employed in healthcare delivery settings. Of the 30 percent, 24 percent were employed in hospitals and 6 percent worked in long-term care facilities and home health care. These demanding environments, where acute patients require intensive services, pose a challenge to recruiting pharmacists. In a 2000 survey conducted by the American Society of Health-System Pharmacists, 44 percent of respondents said their vacancy rates for pharmacists were higher in 2000 than they were five years ago. In terms of recruiting entry-level practitioners, 40 percent of respondents described the overall shortage of pharmacists as "severe," with 70 percent describing the shortage of experienced pharmacists as "severe."

The demand in institutional settings is further intensified by competition for pharmacists trained at the residency or fellowship level. These candidates have more specialized skills, which are needed in the increasingly complex hospital environment.

However, there is a growing gap between the available supply and the real and anticipated demand for pharmacists. The magnitude of this gap is best seen when vacancy rates across healthcare occupations are compared. Vacancy rates in hospitals during 2001 were highest for pharmacists in contrast to other medical and service occupations. The rates were even higher than for nurses, a trend that many healthcare executives may not know.

To compensate for the pharmacist shortage, employers are turning more to pharmacy technicians. According to the *Occupational Outlook Handbook,* employment in this occupation is expected to increase by 21 percent to 35 percent from 2000 to 2010. In 1998, 170,000 pharmacy technician jobs were available, of which 34,000 were in hospitals (U.S. Department of Labor 2002). Technicians supplement the work of the pharmacists by performing routine tasks such as verifying, counting, and labeling prescriptions. In hospitals, they also read patient charts and prepare and deliver medications to patients. Because technicians keep a running inventory of medicines and other supplies, more time is available for pharmacists to talk to patients and manage drug therapies.

There are formal, nonmandatory training programs for technicians that are increasingly favored by employers. However, most of the training is on the job. There are some programs that offer formal pharmacy technician education at locations such as community colleges. The problem is that some technicians never finish these programs because they are hired away by chains and receive on-the-job training. Because most pharmacy technicians receive on-the-job education in all types of employment settings, the level of professionalism and knowledge varies and is specific to the needs of the type of employer.

Where are these trends likely to go? Healthcare organizations will continue to emphasize the roles of technicians to contain costs. Technicians will assume more responsibility for routine tasks previously performed by pharmacists. One constraint is that many states have legislated the maximum number of technicians who can work under a pharmacist. However, because of increased demand for technicians, some states have expanded the allowable ratio of technicians to pharmacists.

At the end of 2001, no pharmacy school in the country had instituted a pharmacy technician program. However, prompted by the shortage of pharmacists, pharmacy technicians can earn formal certification after passing an exam. Some states mandate certification for technicians, and some retail stores gain credibility by requiring it. In most states, the board of pharmacy requires technicians to be registered with state boards, not to mandate educational requirements but to ensure that security measures are upheld. This requirement ensures that a technician who had been a problem at a prior employer, such as for unlawfully dispensing drugs, would be prevented from being hired at another pharmacy.

Advancements in technology, such as machines that automatically dispense medications and computers that instantly verify insurance benefits, can reduce the need for pharmacists in the future. However, demographic patterns certainly point to increased demand. Not surprisingly, recruiting efforts for pharmacists are hampered by the limited supply of these professionals. According to "The Pharmacist Workforce: A Study of the Supply and Demand for Pharmacists" (U.S. Health Resources and Services Administration Bureau of Health Professions 2000a), the number of active pharmacists will actually increase from 196,000 in 2000 to 224,500 in 2010. Although this represents an increase of 14.5 percent, this shows a slowing of the growth in prior years. One reason for this decline is the decrease in pharmacy graduates in the late 1990s. Part of the explanation for this is that all pharmacy schools in the country are transitioning from conferring bachelor of science degrees to doctor of pharmacy (PharmD) degrees. The impact of this change is that it lengthens the educational component and increases the amount of practical experience students should have before moving into the workforce. Most schools had made this transition by 2001, but this transition has required additional faculty and other resources and reduced the

Table 1.4: Pharmacy Program Applications, 1990–1999

Year	Number of Applications (in thousands)	Growth (Decline) from Previous Year
1990	17.7	—
1991	23.3	31.6%
1992	28.9	24.0%
1993	32.9	13.8%
1994	34.2	4.0%
1995	32.7	− 4.4%
1996	33.9	3.7%
1997	29.1	− 14.2%
1998	25.2	− 13.4%
1999	22.8	− 9.5%

Source: Data from "The Pharmacist Workforce: A Study of the Supply and Demand for Pharmacists." 2000. Washington, DC: Government Printing Office.

number of graduates during the conversion time period. Although nine new schools of pharmacy opened between 1980 and 2000, the openings did not substantially increase the number of graduates (U.S. Health Resources and Services Administration Bureau of Health Professions 2000a).

This trend of declining graduations is accompanied by a decrease in applications to pharmacy schools, which were 33 percent lower in 1999 than in 1994. Of course, as fewer students apply for pharmacy school, the pool of potential graduates also declines, which diminishes future supply. Table 1.4 shows the decrease of pharmacy school applications in the last decade.

Declining enrollments is not a universal trend for all degrees. Table 1.5 shows that enrollments did not decrease significantly in all degree-granting programs as it did in nursing programs and pharmacy programs. On the contrary, enrollment for all programs actually increased by 2.9 percent from 1996 to 1999!

Table 1.5: Undergraduate Enrollment in All Degree-Granting Institutions (in thousands)

	Public	Private	Total	Change
1990	9,710	2,250	11,959	—
1991	10,148	2,291	12,439	+4.0%
1992	10,216	2,320	12,537	+ 0.8%
1993	10,012	2,312	12,324	− 1.7%
1994	9,945	2,317	12,263	− 0.5%
1995	9,904	2,328	12,232	− 0.3%
1996	9,935	2,392	12,327	+ 0.8%
1997	10,007	2,443	12,451	+ 1.0%
1998	9,950	2,487	12,437	− 0.1%
1999	10,110	2,571	12,681	+ 2.0%

Source: U.S. Department of Education, National Center for Education Statistics. 2001. "Projections of Education Statistics to 2001." Washington, DC: Government Printing Office.

Allied Health Professionals

Demand for allied health professionals, like the demand for nurses and pharmacists, will also increase according to the *Occupational Outlook Handbook* (U.S. Department of Labor 2000a). Occupational therapists held about 73,000 jobs in 2000, with the largest number employed by hospitals. The number of jobs forecasted through 2010 is expected to grow between 21 percent and 35 percent. Such dramatic growth reflects demographic shifts. Aging baby boomers are likely to require more services as they reach middle age. An increasing population of those 75 years old and older is also more likely to need extensive therapy services to support their activities of daily living. According to these same statistics, there will be an expansion of the school-age population, requiring more occupational therapists to help children with disabilities enter special education programs. These needs will put yet another drain on the available talent pool.

By the same token, the demand for physical therapists should rise by an equivalent amount as a result of the number of individuals with disabilities or limited function requiring physical therapy services (U.S. Department of Labor 2002). There were approximately 132,000 jobs for physical therapists in 2000, and about two-thirds of those were located at hospitals or offices of physical therapists. In addition to the aging baby boom population and rising elderly population, other factors will increase the demand for these professionals. Two critical factors in particular are advances in technology and lifestyle changes. Technological advances, for instance, will save more lives on either end of the life continuum. More trauma victims will also survive because of future medical developments, creating yet additional demand for physical (and occupational) therapy services. In addition, a growing number of employers are using physical therapists for stress reduction and wellness-related programs as well as for injury reduction at the worksite. Such factors account for a projected demand growth of between 21 percent to 35 percent by 2010 (U.S. Department of Labor 2002).

The allied health specialty experiencing even more accelerated growth is respiratory therapy. Respiratory therapists accounted for about 110,000 jobs in 2000, and approximately 80 percent of them served respiratory care, anesthesiology, and pulmonary medicine departments of hospitals. Employment opportunities for respiratory therapists are projected to increase by 21 percent to 35 percent by 2010 (U.S. Department of Labor 2002). These opportunities reflect substantial growth in the middle-aged and elderly sectors of the U.S. population and the increased incidence of cardiopulmonary disease and other debilitating conditions among these groups. As is true for other allied health occupations, the skills of respiratory therapists will be required on an increasing basis to support the technological advances enabling newborns, elderly, and trauma victims to survive.

According to *Career Guide to Industries* (U.S. Department of Labor 2000b), approximately 14 percent of all wage and salary jobs created between 1998 and 2008 are predicted to be in the healthcare industry. In fact, of the 30 fastest growing occupations in the

Table 1.6: Projected Increase in Employment Between 1998 and 2008

Industry/Profession	Growth from 1998 to 2008
All industries	15.3%
Healthcare industry	25.7%
Professional specialty:	
Occupational therapist	30.3%
Pharmacists	11.5%
Physical therapist	34.5%
Registered nurse	21.6%
Respiratory therapist	43.0%

Source: U.S. Department of Labor. 2000. *Career Guide to Industries.* Washington, DC: Government Printing Office.

United States, 12 are in health services. Table 1.6 presents the projected growth rates for various professional specialties in healthcare. As can be seen, most of the growth is expected to exceed that for all other industries.

Service Workers

Service workers are typically responsible for custodial and maintenance services within hospitals. This workforce tends to experience high turnover, as lower-skilled workers move in and out of their positions. According to the American Hospital Association, hospital vacancy rates (see Figure 1.3) for environmental service workers (housekeeping/maintenance) reached 9 percent in 2001 (AHA 2001). Further, of the hospitals that responded to the American Hospital Association's survey in 2001, 24 percent reported they had more difficulty recruiting for these positions than in the previous year. The recruiting problem didn't appear to be the result of salary structures.

Figure 1.3: Vacancy Rates for Selected Hospital Occupations, 2001

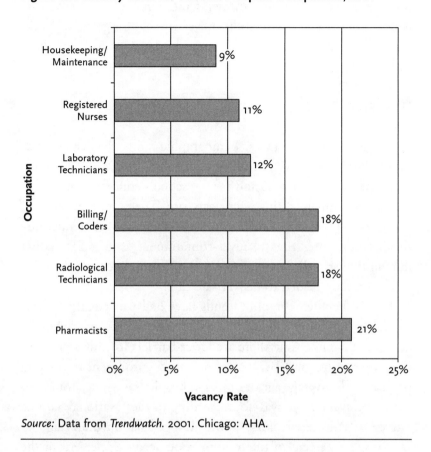

Source: Data from *Trendwatch*. 2001. Chicago: AHA.

According to *Career Guide to Industries* (U.S. Department of Labor 2001), median annual earnings of hospital janitors and cleaners in 1998 were $15,340. In 1997, median annual earnings for these workers in hospitals were $16,800, surpassing other health-care settings except for those owned by the federal government. The same salary pattern is true for supervisors in the field. Median annual earnings for cleaning supervisors were $19,600 in 1998, with corresponding median earnings in hospital settings at

$22,400. It appears that hospitals pay above the norm for this sector of employees. However, throwing more money at the retention issue is not enough to control turnover among this group of workers. Other measures, discussed later in this book, must be in place.

DEMOGRAPHIC TRENDS

Under most circumstances, demographic shifts that create dramatic employment opportunities would be welcome news for employees filling the jobs and for the schools educating the workforce. Unfortunately, this is not the case. There are a number of additional factors associated with these demographic trends, further complicating the turnover-containment issue and feeding into an industry climate that makes it difficult to achieve the minimal retention needed to deliver safe care.

Several key demographic trends have had particularly adverse effects on retention rates. Although the workforce as a whole is aging, at the same time there are fewer barriers for this workforce to leave existing jobs. Because of declining enrollment in nursing programs, the average age of nurses in hospitals is 45, up from 1980 when the average age was 40. According to the "National Sample Survey of Registered Nurses," the RN population under age 30 comprised 9 percent of the total in 2000 versus 25 percent of the total in 1980 (U.S. Health Resources and Services Administration Bureau of Health Professions 2000b). Does an average of five years in age difference really make a difference in retention? Perhaps not if the nature of the work and the work environment remain constant. However, the work and the environment in which that work is delivered have dramatically changed over the years.

As nurses age, the long hours demanded at hospitals become increasingly difficult to endure. The same principle holds true for the demanding physical activities. Older nurses are more susceptible to work-related injuries. Many healthcare workers in this situation find a transition to other jobs that require only eight-hour days (and no weekends) and fewer physical activities particularly attractive. With significant experience behind them, these workers are very appealing to employers in the insurance and pharmaceutical industries. These employers find creative ways to use these workers' skills and greater experience, as we'll see later in this chapter.

By 2010, 40 percent of all RNs will be older than age 50 (U.S. General Accounting Office 2001). With the average age of nurses increasing, many nurses today are closer to retirement age. This, coupled with the decline in enrollment in nursing programs, further constricts the pool of available candidates. To make matters worse, women comprise 94 percent of all RNs. This predominantly female population is often composed of second-wage earners for their household. As a result, many are able to more easily reduce their hours, to separate from their job because of a spousal job transfer, or to quit altogether because they no longer require a second income. In 2000, only 58.5 percent of the total RN population worked full-time in nursing, according to the "National Sample Survey of Registered Nurses" (U.S. Health Resources and Services Administration Bureau of Health Professions 2000b). The Federation of Nurses and Health Professionals (2001) estimated that one out of every five nurses currently working in the healthcare field is considering leaving patient care for reasons other than retirement in the next five years. Given that these projections are not calculated into the labor shortages we're discussing here, the future looks that much bleaker.

These gender dynamics and their implications are not relevant only for nurses. They are likely to affect other healthcare professions as well in the near future. For example, significant reversals in the current gender gap for pharmacists are projected by 2005. Even though pharmacy has traditionally been dominated by men, women will comprise the majority of this profession within the next five years. To illustrate this gender shift, in 1970 women represented 12 percent of active pharmacists (U.S Health Resources and Services Administration 1970–90; 1995–2000). By 2000, women accounted for 46 percent of the pharmacist workforce and are projected to comprise 58 percent of all pharmacists by 2010. There are some very interesting implications of this trend. The Census Bureau's population survey from 1979 to 1998 showed that pharmacists in general worked an average of 41.8 hours per week. However, male pharmacists averaged 44.1 hours per week, while women worked 37.2 hours per week. This means that as women represent a greater proportion of pharmacists, the average number of hours worked per person may well decline, putting additional pressure on staffing requirements.

The other side of the demographic trend is the increasing demand for healthcare services. As baby boomers age, there is a higher demand for hospitals and related services. The number of people over 65 years old will double in the next 30 years. Given the enormity of this demographic age group, there will be significant pressure to increase available health services. This will create significant disparities between the future supply of and demand for caregivers. In terms of pharmaceuticals, the volume of prescription medication is expected to grow from 2.8 billion in 1999 to 3.6 billion in 2004 (U.S. Health Resources and Services Administration Bureau of Health Professions 2000a). This represents a 29 percent increase in the number of prescriptions written, requiring more pharmacists to fill the orders.

Thus, we are faced with cross-trends across multiple professions. The number of available personnel in the workforce is decreasing, while the number of patients who need services is increasing. These demographic trends will continue to put pressure on healthcare organizations to make their work environments both attractive to newcomers and hospitable to current staff members as a way to retain them.

MARKET TRENDS

Another factor adding to the exodus from healthcare delivery is job mobility itself. Today, there is higher job mobility across all

Figure 1.4: Average Total Income of Pharmacists by Employment Setting, 1998

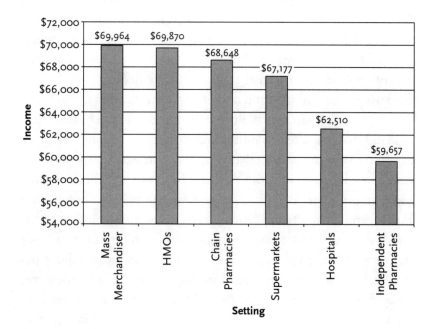

Source: Data from "Drug Topics Salary Surveys." 2000. In *The Pharmacist Workforce: A Study of the Supply and Demand for Pharmacists.* Washington, DC: Government Printing Office.

industries, including in healthcare. Newer workers coming into the workforce are less emotionally committed to the profession than their older counterparts. With more choices and less tolerance for poor working conditions, these workers are exercising their options with their feet, exiting hospitals after two to five years. Other industries are welcoming these healthcare expatriates with open arms.

Pharmacists, for example, have multiple options in employment settings. The majority of pharmacists—over 60 percent—are employed in retail or community settings, where salaries are higher than those offered by their institutional counterparts. Figure 1.4 illustrates the dramatic differences. In 1998, pharmacists' average salaries were almost 12 percent higher in mass-merchandiser settings, such as K-Mart and Wal-Mart, than salaries in hospitals. Given the salary disparity, what is the draw to hospitals? Clearly, for pharmacists, the disparity will continue to increase the attractiveness of employment outside the hospital setting. Abundant job opportunities at more-attractive wage levels will only hasten the exit of qualified pharmacists from healthcare delivery.

This problem is not limited to pharmacists. Low unemployment rates, especially among healthcare workers, coupled with high demand, have resulted in multiple employment options for nurses as well. This trend is exacerbated by the increased competition for experienced nurses, who can pursue jobs in any healthcare setting, including private practices, physician groups, clinics, nursing homes, and rehabilitation centers. Even more threatening to hospitals, however, are the employment opportunities for nurses in other industries. For example, medical device and pharmaceutical companies seek nurses who are skilled in dealing with FDA (Food and Drug Administration)-related clinical issues, particularly those who know how to handle complaints and provide customer satisfaction.

Opportunities abound for nurses in other roles as well, including as insurance company analysts, onsite occupational health nurses, quality assurance reviewers, managed care/HMO analysts, and as technical members of the team that sells or supports the sale of drugs to physicians. With better working conditions, attractive wage levels, and some perceived increase in status, pressures on nurses to leave the delivery arena are significant. Average salaries for nurses also vary by employment setting, as shown in Figure 1.5, making other employment options attractive.

Another market trend that affects retention is the growing criticality of patient satisfaction. In the age of managed care, consumers have choices and many rely on patient satisfaction ratings to select their delivery facility, especially their hospital. This knowledge is increasingly widely dispersed and much more accessible than has been true previously. Consumers of healthcare services are also more demanding, a reflection of their increased

Figure 1.5: Average Total Income of Registered Nurses by Employment Setting, 2001

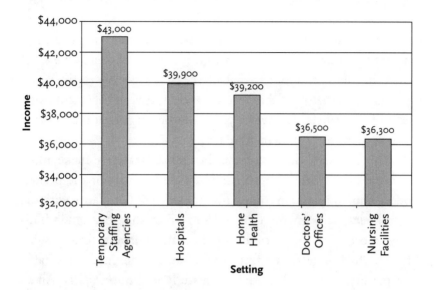

Source: Data from U.S. Department of Labor. 2001. *Occupational Outlook Handbook.* Washington, DC: Government Printing Office, and American Hospital Association. 2001. *Trendwatch.* Chicago: AHA.

sophistication. When receiving services, informed consumers are more likely to practice self-advocacy. This, in turn, places greater demands on healthcare workers, resulting in higher stress, especially in healthcare delivery environments. Where nurses are primary points of patient contact, significant numbers of nurses report job dissatisfaction in large part because of the gap between what they feel they can provide and what they are expected to or should provide. Chronic short staffing creates a self-amplifying situation by intensifying workload for available staff and hence creating more stress and raising their propensity to leave.

Desperate to fill critical vacancies, many hospitals have resorted to offering premium pay in an attempt to lure workers to extend their shifts. Double pay, and in some cases triple pay, has been offered to close short-term staffing gaps. At really difficult times, even this lure is not enough to bring already tired workers back to work. Extended use of travelers, or part-time/temporary staff, is practiced throughout the industry to fill the gaps in staffing. In some noted institutions, traveling staff comprise a significant part of the workforce for great periods of time. One executive in our survey noted that of the 800 RNs his organization employed, over 100 of them were travelers; this arrangement existed to fill vacancies for over a year. Another organization reported that 50 percent of its staff were travelers.

The problem this creates is insidious. Travelers make more money, albeit without benefits. They are not part of the permanent team and have, in some cases, insufficient familiarity with the work being performed on the units to which they're assigned. This puts more, not less, pressure on existing staff and feeds resentment, which negatively affects morale and further intensifies staff's propensity to leave. According to a study in *Health Affairs* (Aiken et al. 2001), more than 40 percent of nurses working in hospitals reported being dissatisfied with their job. Among the reported causes of dissatisfaction were inadequate staffing, increased use of overtime, lack of sufficient support staff, and inadequate wages. Clearly, these market changes lead to a higher propensity for turnover within hospital environments in particular, making an already volatile situation worse.

There are additional pressures on the system brought about by payer action and management response. Funding redesign has also placed significant stress on healthcare workers throughout the industry. Although the number of hospital admissions declined from the mid-1980s to the mid-1990s, they increased between 1995 and 1999. Because funding today only allows patients to stay at the hospital during the most acute portion of their illness, patients who are confined in hospitals have more serious conditions. They are, in essence, too medically complex to be cared for in another setting. With increased acuity of patients and thinner staffing levels because of financial cutbacks throughout the industry, patient-to-caregiver ratios are higher for patients who require extensive attention, further stressing the staff workload and negatively affecting patient outcomes. In addition, shorter lengths of stay allow less time for healthcare workers to develop significant relationships with their patients, undermining the patient experience and staffs' job satisfaction. A study conducted in 1998 and 1999 by University of Pennsylvania researchers revealed that adding another patient to a nurse's workload translates to a 7 percent increase in the likelihood that the patient would die within 30 days of admission. According to Linda Aiken, director of the Center for Health Outcomes and Policy Research at the University of Pennsylvania School of Nursing, "to have more nurses is to have better patient outcomes" (CNN 2002).

To make matters worse, significant restructuring efforts at hospitals have resulted in dramatically increasing the span of control for managers over the last five years or so. All too often, managers have too many direct reports without the necessary supports to manage their workload effectively. This trend heightens the frustration level of incumbent managers and adds to the complexity of managing operations. How much of an impact this has depends on how broad the span of control is. Optimal span-of-control level may vary, from 15 direct reports for each manager to 35 or more direct reports.

In Chapter 7, we will discuss the criteria that dictate optimal levels, which will vary from service to service, unit to unit. It is not uncommon to find 120, and sometimes 200, direct reports for a single manager, which are clearly well above a reasonable limit using any criteria! Job-restructuring efforts have also resulted in mixed success of clinical task reallocation. Some of these initiatives have worked, while others have failed miserably. All attempts have added to the stress and complexity of care delivery. The specific implications of and available remedies for these efforts are discussed in Chapter 7 as well.

Finally, increasing payer pressure makes management infrastructure investment even more difficult to achieve. Insurance companies, primarily concerned with costs, have a vested interest in capturing more services for less money. This puts pressure on healthcare organizations to seek cost efficiencies. As a result, investment in management infrastructure and employee satisfaction have become less of a priority. All of these circumstances converge to increase turnover rates at hospitals and other delivery institutions nationwide.

Against this type of business environment, it's not at all surprising that unionization efforts have increased once again. In 2001, nurses petitioned approximately 150 hospitals to recognize unions; this is three times the number just ten years ago. In 2000, nurses actually struck at 14 hospitals in contrast to 3 in 1996 (McMenamin 2001).The unionization trend is likely to continue in the years ahead. In California, frequently seen as bellwether, approximately 38 percent of all nurses are unionized. Their platform is very clear and focused: unsafe staffing practices (as a result of cost cutting) have created nursing shortages. Until this trend changes, the unions will likely strike a responsive chord with a lot of potential members. The American Nurses Association (ANA), once the organizing arm of the profession, faced competition over the last five years as its state affiliates opted to become independent. In response, ANA created United American Nurses, which joined the AFL-CIO in 2001. Other groups vying for the right to represent nurses are the American Federation of Teachers and the Service Employees International Union.

The clout of these groups shouldn't be underestimated. In California, nurse unions got legislators to regulate the number of patients that nurses can care for safely. Similar laws are being reviewed in at least a dozen other states and in Congress. It appears that the message is if hospital management can't ensure safe patient practices, someone else will (McMenamin 2001). Ironically, a common but self-defeating response by well-intentioned healthcare executives is to throw money at the problem in an attempt to fix it. They give salary increases, recruit internationally, and offer various forms of recruitment and retention bonuses for selected members of the workforce—most notably nurses. The net effect of these efforts has been temporary and has moved a labor pool from one institution to another, as workers jump from one to another to take advantage of available money. Money-based solutions further destabilize the care environment, escalating costs for the organization and alienating those workers who aren't eligible to cash in on bonuses. Sadly, these responses lack an understanding of the underlying root of the problem.

WORK ENVIRONMENT AND ORGANIZATIONAL CULTURE

Organizational culture within the healthcare industry has a crucial and poorly understood impact on retention rates. Historically, strong management cultures have not been prevalent in the healthcare industry. Although other industries have invested in management and process infrastructures for many years, hospitals have only begun to do so within the last decade. Other parts of the delivery system frequently fall behind their hospital counterparts. Since the advent of DRGs, healthcare organizations have been forced to address operational efficiencies to achieve effectiveness. Before then, a "cost-plus" environment papered over inefficiencies that were, in part, a result of poor management infrastructure and the absence of true financial competition and constraint. In sharp contrast, companies such as General Electric, IBM, and Johnson & Johnson have a long-standing history of developing managers and building infrastructure. Even though some healthcare organizations have begun to pursue these activities relatively recently, they do not dedicate as much focus as do their industrial counterparts. Other industries, such as manufacturing, pharmaceuticals, medical device, and technology, place a greater priority on building a clear organizational culture and associated management infrastructure. These efforts are supported by management goals, quantitative objectives, and focused managerial training and development to ensure management accountability for efficient and effective operations.

For various reasons, which we explore in a later chapter, the role of the manager is still inadequately understood and consequently undervalued in healthcare. The systematic development of management has not attained the same attention in healthcare that it receives elsewhere. Training budgets for managers are typically lower in healthcare organizations than in their industrial counterparts. For example, in other industries training requirements for all employees typically exceed 2 percent of their working time. For managers, this job-related development may encompass two to four weeks of time or more, occupying 4 percent to 8 percent of working time. This substantial investment in training supports management infrastructure and provides tools for the effective management and development of staff. In healthcare, investment in management development has lagged behind other areas deemed more "relevant" to the delivery of patient care.

One significant investment that has been made is in the non-managerial ranks of nursing. "Shared governance," as it has been referred to, has had a very interesting impact on organizational performance. As a concept, shared governance is unique to the healthcare industry, and within the industry it is unique to nursing. Once the rage in the late 1980s and through the early 1990s, shared governance, partners in practice, and similar models are being actively called into question or are dying on the vine. Implicitly, shared governance was an attempt to loosen nursing management's grip on the workforce. Explicitly, it was an attempt to broaden nursing staff's participation in decision making, which is itself a noble goal. Critics of shared governance at the time were drowned out in the din of its popularity. In retrospect, it was actually an overreaction to a dysfunctional management structure and philosophy that clearly needed to change.

Ironically, shared governance's management philosophy, intricate design, formal and complex process, and unrealistic expectations from staff converged to replace one dysfunctional management structure with yet another. Promising broad collaboration, improved decision making, critical thinking skills, and increased identification with organizational goals, it delivered substantially less than it promised. It also became exceedingly expensive at a time when hospitals needed to dramatically reduce costs. (Extended meetings do not come cheaply and take clinical staff away from the bedside.) In its wake, shared governance may have left more serious problems than it addressed. In the process of instituting shared governance, staff expectations about autonomy and peer review were inflated. This fed the perspective that managers were essentially irrelevant except as keepers of the budget. With "self-scheduling" increasing in popularity, allowing staff to do what they wanted became the path of least resistance. Confused, managers hunkered down or joined the staff who were mobilizing against new cost controls imposed by senior management.

Given the inherent problems of the shared governance model, what accounts for its widespread appeal and broad implementation? Is there something about the profession and its preparation that would make so many gravitate to this model? Some historical reflection may prove useful in answering the question. In the late 1970s, the senior author of this book was told the following story by a group of nurses for whom she was conducting a session on the expanded role of nursing. The discussion was about why it was particularly difficult for nurses to challenge the status quo. The explanation was imbedded in the following anecdote: In nursing school, the first-year students (as a group) stood for the second-year students, who in turn stood for the third-year students, who stood for the instructor, who also stood when a physician walked in. This anecdote represents nursing's strong sense of place, of structure, of rules, and of hierarchy.

With the advantage of hindsight, historical emphases on rigid structures may have led innovators to overengineer the process of engaging nursing staff, prescribing unit council structures, division councils, etc., using a formal labyrinth of rules and groups that ran outside the hospital's line-reporting structure. Was it inadvertent that the structures undermined managerial effectiveness? Or was it perhaps purposive? Or it just may have taken a strong countervailing force to loosen the autocratic management structures that were more normative in the field at the time. Today, remnants of strong preferences for structure and rules do come out, sometimes in unusual ways. Take, for instance, repeated requests by nurses for structuring collaboration and decision making: "Now, exactly what decisions will I be able to make and will the others know I'll be making them?" Working through the gray areas efficiently and developing consensus around such conceptual issues have been a challenge across the board.

Complicating this situation is the fact that clinicians are trained technically to take care of people. With few exceptions, clinicians are not professionally prepared to become managers without training. In other industries, such as those dominated by engineers, the investment is more likely to be made to enable these "technical" employees to become effective managers.

Today, cultural factors—most notably, investment in management infrastructure—have a significant bearing on recruitment and retention. However, the extent of the vulnerability caused by the absence of such infrastructure is not widely understood. Historically, hospitals had been able to thrive despite their inefficiencies and lack of attention to conventional management issues. Third-party insurers over time only exacerbated this problem. Throughout the 1980s and early 1990s, medical procedures were only reimbursed if they had to be done in the hospital. This is clearly not a policy designed to improve efficiency and lower cost.

With the introduction of prospective payment and the Balanced Budget Act, hospitals were forced to reduce their expenses. Because the cost of building and maintaining a management infrastructure was by and large not a part of the cost structure, the argument for investing in it since the cost pressures have been on has not been well received. However, this lack of a management infrastructure remains the chokepoint for an industry that desperately requires the systematic engagement of its well-intentioned human resources in goal-directed, efficient, and effective problem solving. If healthcare executives didn't invest in building the infrastructure when they could, they are loathe to make the investment now when margins are razor thin, if there are margins at all. Yet it is in this very investment that the solutions to these complex issues of recruitment and retention lie.

CONCLUSION

The human resource crisis in healthcare looms large. Shortages of workers throughout the industry have escalated during the 1990s, and we expect them to continue into the foreseeable future. Turnover rates in the industry only exacerbate the problem of a declining labor pool across all healthcare professions. To deal effectively with the crisis, the mandate for healthcare executives is to introduce creative recruitment strategies, increase retention rates, and contain turnover. Solutions require an understanding of the factors underlying current trends, such as changes in demographics, market conditions, and healthcare financing and the dynamics of organizational culture.

Together these trends have set in motion a series of events that resulted in chronic short staffing. This, in turn, creates a self-amplifying situation, intensifying workloads for available staff that create more stress, raise their propensity to leave, and yield negative health outcomes. Against the background of historically limited investment in infrastructure and unwieldy managerial spans of control, limited financial resources make such investment difficult but no less essential. For healthcare executives serious about addressing the underlying causes of today's recruitment and retention issues the answer lies in such investment to build an effective management infrastructure.

REFERENCES

ACT. 1997–2001. "National Reports; Distribution of Planned Educational Majors and ACT Composite Scores." [Online information]. www.act.org.

Aiken L. H., S. P. Clarke, D. M. Sloane, J. A. Sochalski, R. Busse, H. Clarke, P. Giovannetti, J. Hunt, A. M. Rafferty, and J. Shamian. 2001. "Nurses' Reports on Hospital Care in Five Countries." *Health Affairs* 20 (3): 43–53.

American Association of Colleges of Nursing. 2000. "2000–2001 Enrollment and Graduations in Baccalaureate and Graduate Programs in Nursing." Washington, DC: American Association of Colleges of Nursing.

American Hospital Association. 2001. *Trendwatch.* Chicago: American Hospital Association.

American Society of Health-System Pharmacists. 2000. "ASHP Survey Reveals Increase in Open Positions at Hospital and Health-System Pharmacies." [Online information; retrieved 9/02]. www.ashp.com/news/showarticle.cfm.

Buerhaus, P., D. Auerbach, and D. O. Staiger. 2000. "Implications of an Aging Registered Nurse Workforce." *Journal of the American Medical Association* 282: 2948–54.

Bureau of National Affairs. 2001. "Job Absence and Turnover." *Bulletin to Management* [online publication, volume 10 and 37]. www.bna.com.

CNN. 2000. [Online article; retrieved 10/23/02]. www.cnn.com/2002/health/10/23/nurse.staffing.ap

Federation of Nurses and Health Professionals. 2001. "The Nurse Shortage: Perspective from Current Direct Care Nurses and Former Direct Care Nurses." Latham, NY: New York State United Teachers.

Hospital & Healthcare Compensation Service. 2001. "Hospital Salary and Benefits Report, 2000–2001." [Online information; retrieved 10/02]. www.hhcsinc.com.

McMenamin, B. 2001. "Here We Go Again." *Forbes* (November 12): 48.

U.S. Congressional Research Service. 2001. "CRS Report for Congress. A Shortage of Registered Nurses: Is It On the Horizon or Already Here?" Washington, DC: Government Printing Office.

U.S. Department of Education, National Center for Education Statistics. 2001. "Projections of Education Statistics to 2001." Washington, DC: Government Printing Office.

U.S. Department of Health and Human Services, National Council on Nurse Education and Practice. 1996. Washington, DC: Government Printing Office.

U.S. Department of Labor. 2000a. *Occupational Outlook Handbook.* Washington, DC: Government Printing Office.

———. 2000b. *Career Guide to Industries.* Washington, DC: Government Printing Office.

———. 2001. *Career Guide to Industries.* Washington, DC: Government Printing Office.

———. 2002. *Occupational Outlook Handbook.* Washington, DC: Government Printing Office.

U.S. General Accounting Office. 2001. "Nursing Workforce: Emerging Nurse Shortages Due to Multiple Factors." GAO-01–944. Washington, DC: General Accounting Office.

U.S. Health Resources and Services Administration. 1970–90. "Factbook." Washington, DC: Government Printing Office.

U.S. Health Resources and Services Administration Bureau of Health Professions. 1995–2000. "Pharmacist Supply Model." Washington, DC: Government Printing Office.

———. 2000a. "The Pharmacist Workforce: A Study of the Supply and Demand for Pharmacists." Washington, DC: Government Printing Office.

———. 2000b. "National Sample Survey of Registered Nurses." Washington, DC: Government Printing Office.

CHAPTER 2

The Role of Measurement
and Accountability

HISTORICALLY THE MEASUREMENT of turnover (when it was measured) used to be the responsibility of someone in human resources—not necessarily a particular person with a particular title, just someone within the department. In an industry where people joined a profession, identified strongly with it, and tended to stay for their entire careers, the problem of turnover in healthcare was a relative nonissue. Thus, there was little perceived value for systematic approaches to measuring turnover to understand and control it. The real problem of turnover—people voluntarily leaving their positions and the organization for something else—is a relatively new concern for healthcare organizations.

Only recently has turnover begun to receive the systematic attention it so richly deserves. Even now, surprisingly few institutions have the measurement apparatus to really get a handle on the problem. As a result of less-than-optimal measurement, we're left with only a gross understanding of the problem and no one to hold accountable for its resolution. Trying to solve a problem as complex and important as turnover with gross solutions won't work, in the same way that treating a specific infection with a nonspecific antibiotic won't eliminate the infection. Effective measurement of turnover allows surgically precise intervention. If we know the specific characteristics of the individuals (or groups) that are at risk for leaving at a given point in their tenure with the facility we can develop specifically targeted retention strategies to retard mass exits as well as prevent the propensity to leave in the first place.

SURVEYING THE TOP-100 HOSPITALS

Given the criticality of recruitment, retention and turnover to the future of healthcare, Numerof & Associates, Inc. (NAI) conducted a survey in the spring of 2000 to gather data in four primary areas that most directly affect retention and turnover:

1. Turnover rates and trends
2. Measurement and accountability for managing turnover
3. Retention methods and effectiveness
4. Future initiatives

This chapter focuses on the first two areas—(1) turnover rates and trends and (2) measurement and accountability for managing turnover. The results of the survey are eye opening and have significant implications for practical application throughout the industry.

Starting with "the best in class," NAI selected the top 100 hospitals in the United States to participate in the survey. Rated by Solucient Leadership Institute (formerly HCIA-SACHs), an organization that provides strategic healthcare information and market intelligence and analysis, these hospitals achieved their high marks based on assessments of clinical quality, operational efficiency, and financial health. Vice presidents and directors of human resources at the identified hospitals received the initial survey questionnaire, and follow-up actions consisted of an additional mailing and phone calls to encourage participation.

Thirty-eight hospitals participated in the written survey and another 30 participated in structured interviews, for a 68 percent

Figure 2.1: Composition of Respondent Hospitals, by Geographic Region

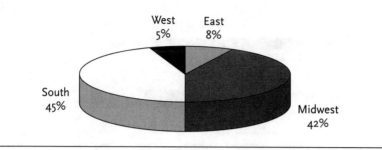

overall response rate. No meaningful differences between survey and interview respondents were observed. In light of this, discussion of the two groups is combined. Respondent hospitals had an average of 2,882 employees, with actual numbers ranging from 170 to 10,000. In addition, these hospitals had an average of 422 beds, with actual numbers ranging from 30 beds to 1,200 beds. Geographic factors were also considered for the survey. Of those surveyed, 29 percent classified their hospital as located in an urban setting, 45 percent in a suburban setting, and 26 percent in a rural setting. In addition, 76 percent of the hospitals identified themselves as a community hospital while the remaining 24 percent classified their hospital as a teaching institution. The geographical dispersion of respondent hospitals is depicted in Figure 2.1.

TURNOVER RATES AND TRENDS

Responding administrators were asked what their staff turnover rates had been over the last three years. The aggregate turnover rate for survey participants increased from almost 19 percent in 1997 to almost 21 percent in 1999 (see Figure 2.2). Consistent with national data for healthcare turnover cited earlier, this represents less than a 1 percent increase per year. When categorized by setting, urban hospitals experienced a slightly larger increase, while suburban hospitals

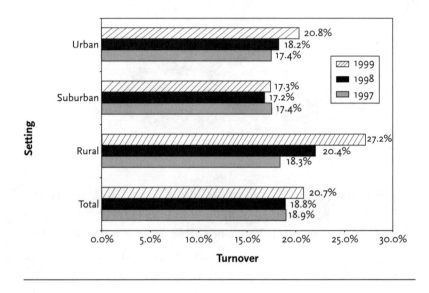

actually remained steady during the period. However, rural hospitals experienced significant increases in turnover rates from 1997 to 1999, when turnover reached a staggering 27 percent. Even though the turnover rate in rural hospitals was only slightly higher than in other geographic settings in 1997, they suffered an aggregate increase of 3.5 percent between 1997 and 1998 and an aggregate increase of 5.5 percent between 1998 and 1999.

Next, respondents were surveyed about their own perceptions of turnover trends within their hospital. Over half (59 percent) of aggregate respondents felt that turnover was increasing at their respective hospital, consistent with the actual data. Another 9 percent suggested it was on the decline, while 26 percent felt no change over the time period. Six percent were unsure about whether or not any change had occurred. However, when classified by hospital setting, only 38 percent of rural hospital respondents perceived that turnover was increasing during the three-year period, and 22 percent did not know whether their turnover was increasing. This is inconsistent with actual industry trends, which

Figure 2.3: Attention to Retention, by Geographic Setting

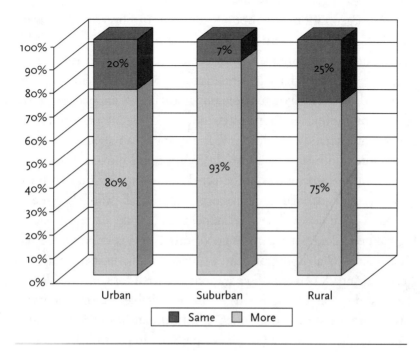

clearly indicate that turnover in rural hospitals dramatically increased.

Eighty-five percent of all respondents also reported that they were devoting more attention to the retention issue than they had in the past. This figure is slightly lower at rural hospitals, where 75 percent reported that they were devoting more attention to retention than they had previously (see Figure 2.3). Ironically 93 percent of suburban hospitals, where turnover rates had been stable, reported devoting more attention to the issue. Interestingly, rural hospitals were experiencing higher turnover, were less aware of it, and devoted less attention to it than their suburban and urban counterparts. Rural institutions must clearly focus more resources on addressing turnover- and retention-related issues.

These findings are quite telling in that any efforts to manage turnover require an understanding of it. Clearly, hospitals must first develop a realistic picture of their own situation to effectively address their retention issues.

As organizations attempt to confront turnover issues, distinguishing between controllable separations versus uncontrollable separations is important. Controllable separations consist of those reasons to leave that, if circumstances were different, may be reversed. These include such reasons as leaving for an increase in pay, better promotional opportunities, or a better working environment. These are certainly conditions that a hospital can affect, which will therefore minimize separations. In contrast, uncontrollable turnover reflects those separations not affected by the organization itself but by objective external circumstances such as relocation because of spousal job transfer, illness, retirement, and death.

When asked what percentage of turnover was controllable versus uncontrollable, respondents assigned fairly even percentages to each, citing 48 percent of separations occurred for controllable reasons and 52 percent occurred for uncontrollable reasons. However, as Figure 2.4 shows, respondents from urban hospitals attributed more of their turnover (almost 54 percent) to controllable factors, whereas respondents from rural hospitals had the opposite response. Rural institutions attributed only 36.5 percent of their turnover to controllable factors and a significant majority (63.5 percent) of their separations to uncontrollable factors. This may provide a rationale for why rural hospitals devoted less attention to turnover than their urban and suburban counterparts. If they didn't perceive their turnover as controllable, they may have believed that there was little they could do to positively affect the situation.

MEASUREMENT AND ACCOUNTABILITY
FOR MANAGING TURNOVER

Respondents were also asked whether they measured turnover on a regular basis. As a group, 89 percent of the hospitals in the study measured turnover regularly. When broken down by setting, how-

Figure 2.4: Controllable Versus Noncontrollable Turnover, by Geographic Setting

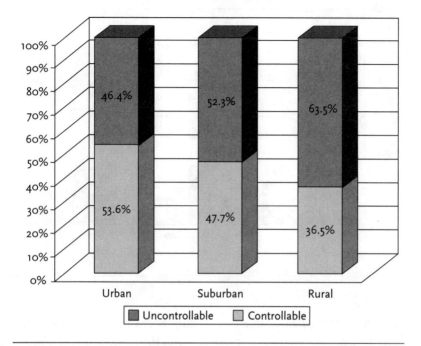

ever, we begin to see some industry differences (see Figure 2.5). All of the suburban hospitals measured turnover, and more than half of those reported it on a monthly basis. Ninety percent of urban hospitals measured turnover, and most reported quarterly or annually. However, only two-thirds of rural hospitals measured turnover, and half of those did so on a quarterly basis. This suggests that rural hospitals were not taking as analytical of an approach to this issue as their suburban counterparts in particular, but they were experiencing the biggest problem.

Does regular measurement actually affect turnover? Do we see a difference in average turnover rates depending on whether or not turnover is being measured? Is it possible that those hospitals that were measuring turnover on a regular basis tended to have lower turnover rates than those that did not measure it regularly? If so,

Figure 2.5: Frequency of Calculating Turnover Statistics

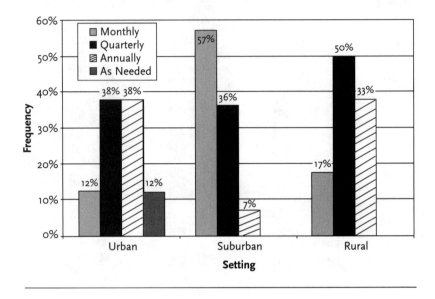

this does point to a possible relationship between measurement and actual turnover experience. Logically, to effectively manage a problem, one must be aware of the existence and extent of the problem. In measuring it regularly, we may be more likely to do something about it. However, turnover cannot really be addressed systematically unless defined measurable objectives related to turnover are in place. When asked if their hospitals had developed quantifiable objectives to measure turnover, only 32 percent indicated they had established some objectives. However, of those institutions, only a little more than half defined a quantifiable retention rate as a goal (see Figure 2.6). For those hospitals that had quantifiable goals, their goals were very clear and included the following:

- Decrease voluntary turnover to 15 percent by year 2010
- Achieve turnover rates at least 2 percentage points lower than the Bureau of National Affairs's national healthcare rate
- Reduce controllable turnover to 8 percent

Figure 2.6: Reported Use of Retention Objectives

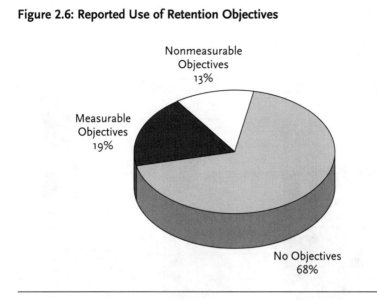

Nonmeasurable Objectives 13%

Measurable Objectives 19%

No Objectives 68%

Nonquantifiable objectives included:

- Conduct reviews during initial assessment period to establish areas of needs
- Incorporate retention goals into employee satisfaction
- Incorporate retention goals into performance appraisals

The hospitals' likelihood of attaching measurable objectives to retention was influenced by setting (see Figure 2.7). Although only 22 percent of rural hospitals set objectives, a proportionately higher number of urban and suburban hospitals established these objectives. In fact, for two out of three urban hospitals that established retention objectives, the objectives were quantifiable.

The mere fact that turnover was being measured at all may have had some interesting impacts. In general, turnover rates were lower for those hospitals in the survey that had measurable, quantifiable objectives, providing further evidence that merely paying attention to the problem of turnover may influence its outcomes. Beyond this,

Figure 2.7: Use of Measurable Retention Objectives, by Geographic Setting

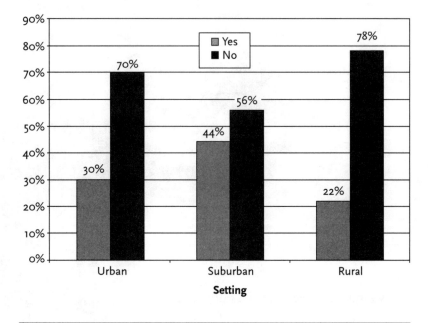

defining a specific quantifiable goal to determine whether turnover is within acceptable limits is a critical strategy in the management of turnover. In addition to passively influencing the outcomes, measurement helps to determine whether and to what extent the hospital should pursue aggressive remediation strategies.

Addressing retention effectively also requires an organization to understand which management level will have the most impact on turnover and to measure trends accordingly. In the case of respondent hospitals, 47 percent indicated that they calculated turnover based on more discreet levels such as by department, unit, or supervisor (see Figure 2.8). Perhaps most importantly, of the 47 percent that measured turnover at more than a gross organizational level, 21 percent calculated turnover statistics by unit or below. Retention by department level—or more desirably, by unit level—is a critical

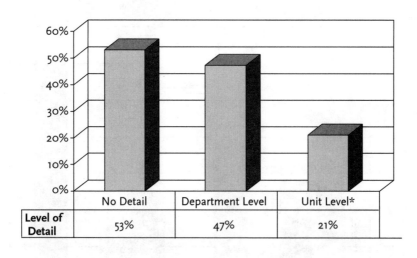

Level of Detail	No Detail	Department Level	Unit Level*
	53%	47%	21%

data point based on our own healthcare experience and research. Managers have a significant impact on employee retention that correlates strongly to turnover at the unit level. An employee's issue with his or her manager contributes substantially to the probability of his or her leaving the organization, because day-to-day contact has a profound impact on staff. In support of this concept, one hospital indicated that its quantitative turnover objectives were established at the departmental level. It is noteworthy that none of the hospitals established quantitative objectives at the unit level.

As Figure 2.9 shows, 28 percent of those hospitals that measured turnover by department calculated results at least quarterly, and another 39 percent calculated results on an as-needed basis. In contrast, hospitals that measured turnover at the unit level were less likely to report it on a quarterly or more-frequent basis (37 percent combined) and more likely to do so on an as-needed basis (62 percent).

Understanding which management level most clearly affects turnover is one thing. Holding people accountable for managing

Figure 2.9: Frequency of Calculation, by Management Level

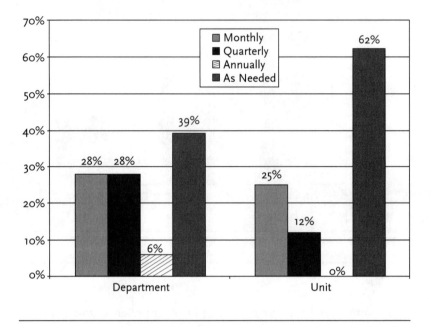

turnover once it is measured is another. To understand this, the survey also explored who within the organization was actually held accountable for retention. Historically, accountability for managing turnover within hospitals had been with the human resources department and was managed at the gross level. As noted earlier, management accountability at the first or second line of management greatly influences turnover behavior. When asked who was accountable for managing retention, only one-half (50 percent) of the respondents indicated that it was the responsibility of department managers or below. In addition, 13 percent also held senior managers accountable (see Figure 2.10). This latter level does have an impact, albeit to a lesser degree than department managers, on whether employees leave. The fact that they were held accountable, however, suggests that they would be more engaged with their managers in creating an environment more conducive to

Figure 2.10: Who Is Accountable for Retention?

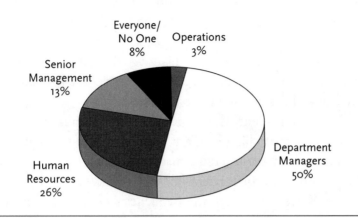

retention. In addition, 26 percent of respondents continued to hold human resources accountable for gross retention, which had little impact. A couple of respondents noted that within their organization, human resources was charged with providing the tools to facilitate and improve retention but that line managers were ultimately responsible for the results. This is a reasonable division of accountability. Finally, 8 percent of the hospitals reported that everyone was accountable, with no one in particular charged with the responsibility. Ironically, this underscores the notion that if everyone is responsible, no one is really responsible.

How did accountability trends vary by setting? When examined by setting, half of urban hospitals and a slightly greater number of suburban hospitals held department managers accountable for retention. In sharp contrast, less than half of rural hospitals did so. Given the correlation between holding department managers accountable for retention and lower turnover rates, which was noted earlier, it is surprising that so few organizations take the extra time and effort to measure and hold managers accountable by department. However, merely saying that we hold managers accountable for turnover by itself does not effectively promote retention. Measures for ensuring accountability and rewarding managers for their retention performance must be implemented to ensure that retention remains a top priority. Of the 50 percent of hospitals that placed retention responsibility with department managers, only 29 percent of them actually enforced standards based on definitive criteria (see Figure 2.11). Thus, many hospitals held their department managers accountable but had no formal mechanism for enforcing these measures.

Of the 29 percent who actually measured management's performance in controlling turnover, more than one-half incorporated a retention target into the actual performance-appraisal process. Others indicated that retention was connected with year-end bonuses. Listed below are the frequencies of responses for using particular accountability mechanisms.

Mechanisms for Management Accountability	Respondents Who Used the Tool
Performance appraisal	18.4%
Satisfaction measures of employees	11.0%
On-time performance reviews for employees	5.3%
Bonus is dependent on retention goals	2.6%
Attendance at monthly leadership training	2.6%
Compliance with compensation plan	2.6%

THE FOCUS OF RETENTION

Gross indicators of turnover, even when unit managers are held accountable, are not nearly as effective as targeted indicators such as tenure, position, and related key demographic factors. How were retention efforts focused on specific groups in the hospitals in this study? When asked if hospitals focused their retention efforts on particular job groups, two-thirds of respondents indicated they did. Analyzed by setting, 90 percent of urban hospitals focused their efforts on particular job groups, 73 percent of suburban hospitals did so, and only 25 percent of rural hospitals focused efforts.

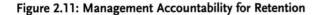

Figure 2.11: Management Accountability for Retention

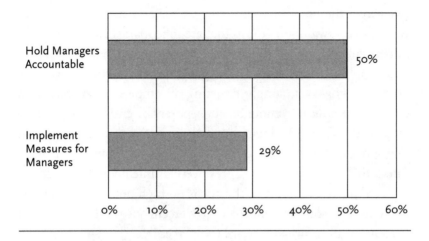

When identifying the job groups on which respondents concentrated their retention efforts, an overwhelming number (55 percent) targeted nursing staff. Focusing on nurses is logical because these positions account for the majority of hospital employees. However, it is what is not focused on that is problematic. Only 24 percent of the hospitals focused on pharmacists, and still fewer focused on other at-risk occupations. Thirteen percent geared efforts toward information technology employees and a corresponding percentage focused on allied health professionals. Given the critical shortages of these other occupations, the lack of attention to focused turnover management is striking. Further, nurses, pharmacists, and allied health professionals are front-line staff and must be accessible to patients. A shortage of these categories of staff will adversely affect patient care.

Traditionally, hospitals have been more reactive to retention issues than organizations in other industries. However, some hospitals are slower to react than others. For example, even in this study of the top-100 institutions several respondents indicated that they began to focus retention efforts on pharmacists only after a shortage of pharmacists emerged. The same principle holds true for other professional groups and geographic areas. To manage the manpower crisis, hospitals and delivery institutions must be proactive across the board in identifying trends and customizing retention efforts toward job groups that are in jeopardy. Rural hospitals, in particular, are more vulnerable because there is frequently a limited supply of labor within close geographical proximity to those hospitals. However, simply targeting all employees for retention efforts is simply not enough. High-potential employees must be identified. When asked whether retention efforts were focused on high-potential employees, only 36 percent of all respondents indicated that customized measures were implemented to address these employees. Ironically, this focus on high potentials was more likely to take place in suburban (40 percent) or rural hospitals (38 percent) than in urban settings (20 percent).

Although industries in general focus on top performers in multiple positions across the organization, healthcare traditionally focuses on those positions that comprise the bulk of the workforce—that is, nurses. Although this makes sense from a staffing standpoint, such unitary focus is shortsighted. Resources must be devoted to all key positions and to identifying top employees, focusing retention efforts on them as well regardless of job category. Such broadening will clearly support the development of a viable management infrastructure discussed in Chapter 1.

CONCLUSION

In part because the problem of turnover has been a relatively new phenomenon in the healthcare industry, it has only recently begun to receive the systematic attention it so richly deserves. Unfortunately, surprisingly few institutions have the measurement tools to actively understand and manage it with the precision that is required.

Results of NAI's 2000 survey of top-100 hospitals yielded some interesting findings. Rural hospitals, who actually experienced higher turnover than their suburban and urban counterparts, were less aware of and devoted less attention to the problem than suburban and urban hospitals. Urban hospitals were more likely than either suburban or rural hospitals to describe their turnover as controllable. Although most of the hospitals (89 percent) surveyed measured turnover regularly, only 32 percent actually developed measurable objectives related to turnover. Given that turnover cannot really be addressed systematically unless defined measurable objectives are in place, this finding clearly pinpoints a vulnerability for hospitals. The mere fact that turnover was being measured may have had some interesting impacts. In general, turnover rates were lower for those surveyed hospitals that had measurable, quantifiable objectives.

However, none of the hospitals established quantitative objectives at the unit level. Yet at the unit level is where managers can have the greatest impact on turnover. Equally important is how organizations held managers accountable for retention. Our findings here are troubling. Many hospitals that held department managers "accountable" for retention had no formal mechanism for enforcing these measures. Finally, we learned that although hospitals tended to zero-in on nursing turnover trends within their institutions, few addressed other at-risk groups but needed to do so.

CHAPTER 3

Commonly Used
Retention Methods

ONE OF THE purposes for the retention survey was to understand which retention methods were being used in the top-100 hospitals and, even more importantly, to determine which of these retention methods were perceived as most and least effective among these hospitals. This chapter explores what is being done to retain staff and examines which methods might be more appropriate under different circumstances.

Respondents were asked to identify those retention methods they typically used in their hospitals. Twenty-seven different and distinct "retention methods" were identified by survey participants. These methods fall into several clusters, as seen in Table 3.1. Some very interesting patterns emerge when we explore the issues associated with each of these clusters. Not surprisingly compensation, benefits, and training/development comprise the bulk of methods employed to address retention issues. The effectiveness of each method is a separate question and is explored later in this chapter. What is important to note is that although many of these methods were frequently used and believed to be effective, they were ultimately not and some in fact were self-defeating.

Table 3.1: Retention Methods, by Cluster

	Respondents Who Used the Method
Compensation	
Compensation reviews/increases	57%
Discretionary/individual salary adjustments	38%
Retention bonuses	35%
Benefits	
Upgrade the health plan	30%
Tuition reimbursement/educational assistance	30%
Upgrade the retirement/pension plan	24%
Flexible benefits	19%
Training and Development	
Management development training	51%
Training in new techniques/equipment	35%
Cross-training opportunities	30%
Cultural diversity programs	24%
Management Access and Communication	
Broad forums for top-management access	57%
Employee-issues hotline	41%
Top-management attendance at staff meetings	38%
Employee suggestion program	27%
Generally "enhance" communication	5%
Career Development/Internal Promotion	
Career-development information	22%
Preference to internal promotion	11%
Scheduling	
Flexible scheduling	55%
Ease of internal transfers	19%
Recognition	
Hospital-branded merchandise	42%
Recognition programs	11%
Celebrations and institutionwide events	5%
Task Forces and Employee Surveys	
Employee surveys	58%
Retention task force—hospital level	51%
Retention task force—system level	24%
Staffing	
Address staffing and span of control	11%

ZEROING IN ON RETENTION METHODS

Compensation and Benefits

Most of the institutions that used more frequent compensation reviews and increases did so as needed, with 25 percent of them ensuring that it was done at least twice a year. Retention bonuses and discretionary adjustments typically occurred as needed. Across industries, management has attempted, for decades, to shape employee behavior with money and benefits, despite what research has consistently shown. Put simply, money and benefits, assuming internal and external equity for given positions, are important "basic satisfiers." They do not motivate behavior over the long term, even though all of us would like more money! Management typically places more importance on these factors than their employees do.

In healthcare today, the problems associated with not fully understanding this behavioral dynamic are quite significant. Healthcare organizations, desperate to secure clinical talent short term have been vying with others for this scarce workforce. Starting with nurses, they've offered signing bonuses as a recruitment device followed by retention bonuses as a measure to hold on to the staff they've bought. Essentially, these staff members become long-term temps, loyal to the money but not to the institution that recruited them. Only during the Y2K crisis with IT professionals has this type of lure been used on a mass basis.

Signing bonuses have long been used very selectively to bring on special individual talent typically at senior management levels. The implications of this for the industry are just now beginning to unfold, and we predict they will have long-term and very serious negative consequences. We see nurses staying at one institution just long enough to cash in before moving on to the next bonus. Because many of these institutions did not anticipate the "jump ship" phenomenon, they designed lures with short-term incentives. Neighboring institutions who may not have wanted to (or needed to) play the money game found that they had little choice but to join in to attract new graduates. As one noted and insightful healthcare human resources executive put it, "When these hospitals increase their incentives to attract workers, all they do is increase the industry's total cost of delivering care. Everyone else raises and meets the new salary levels; the total market goes up, but it doesn't address any of the fundamental problems."

The bigger issue is that other employee groups have joined the compensation game. Once defended as a legitimate response to market demands and shortages, non-nurses are now making their voices heard loudly. It's their turn to shout "market demand" and internal "inequity." And many of them appear to be quite successful, as noted in Chapter 1, especially pharmacists and a variety of allied health professionals including therapists of all types. Perhaps the most serious problem with compensation and benefits as responses to such systemic issues as described in Chapter 1 is that even though they don't fix the problem they're very difficult to take back once given out.

Compensation strategy is formulated in the context of the whole competitive picture—that is, the power of your brand, your image and reputation, your facilities, etc. A strong competitive position can allow an organization to set its salary price point slightly below market from a policy point of view. The attractiveness of the organization itself, assuming that it is effectively communicated, would be relied on to provide the differential. This assumes too that there is sufficient flexibility to ensure that highly competitive offers can be made to specific individuals when the circumstances are appropriate. The discount that is thus possible—up to about 8 percent— offsets some of the costs associated with building a positive and distinctive work environment. Leveraged across the workforce on an annual basis, this can be a significant savings.

Training and Development

The range of activities implied by training and development reflects actions that are critical to running an organization under any circumstances. The fact that these are defined as retention approaches or "methods" speaks to the lack of investment in infrastructure noted in Chapter 1. Management development training, as noted by survey respondents, referred to training focused on increasing management's awareness of retention issues, turnover data, and recruitment activity. Clearly, this can convey important information, but it's not a method to affect retention systematically. Similarly, training in new techniques/equipment is absolutely necessary to do the job and do it safely. But as a retention tool or method? Unlikely. These interventions are critical just to stay in the game.

Cross-training opportunities begin to get at job development issues, which, in fact, have a bearing on staff's value and flexibility and an institution's ability to staff safely. If done well, cross-training can add to staff identification with the work. If not done well, staff will feel "pulled" into areas of less comfort, harking back to the days of unit rotation, which is a major job dissatisfier for many staff—most clearly nurses.

Finally, cultural diversity programs, to the extent that they help ethnically or culturally diverse staff groups to communicate more effectively and actually solve complex problems constructively, can go far in improving the work climate. Most of these programs, however, provide "awareness" only. Program attendees typically go back to their work areas without the skills to help them work through their differences, and most managers have neither the time, span of control, nor skills to help them.

Management Access and Communication

The activities involved in management access and communication create opportunities for employees to have exposure to senior management. Here, too, the approaches described by survey respondents were all reasonable management responses under normal circumstances. They reflect good management practices at the organizational level. But to see these as adequate responses to the problem of retention is another issue. For example, forums for top-management access included town hall meetings, "meet the CEO" breakfasts, etc. As communication vehicles that provide insight into issues, they should be part of every organization's standard operating procedures. Similarly, "employee-issues hotlines" or "President's hotlines," as they are called in some organizations, are critical real-time links to the issues that concern employees. Most of these connect directly to the CEO's office or to human resources and allow callers to remain anonymous. To the extent that these vehicles, along with suggestion programs, are used to identify trends, resolve specific issues, and demonstrate responsiveness to concerns, they are important tools and should be in place. It's noteworthy that relatively few institutions in our survey had these elements as part of their infrastructure. But, even so, they should not be considered retention methods.

Career Development/Internal Promotion

Providing employees with information about future career opportunities links employees' individual goals with the broader goals and objectives of the organization. To the extent that available information is translated into legitimate career paths for employees, retention goals are indeed served. Although only 22 percent of respondents promoted career development information systematically, even fewer (11 percent) gave preference to internal candidates when promotion opportunities occurred. Ironically, those who gave preferential treatment to internal, qualified candidates reported that it was their single most-effective retention tool.

Scheduling

A surprising 55 percent of respondents used flexible scheduling as a recruitment and retention tool. Given the criticality of bringing qualified staff into the organization, many healthcare organizations have used scheduling options to enable staff flexibility. This practice has gotten out of hand for some hospitals, as employees became accustomed to literally working when they wanted to rather then when the facility needed them! Going "casual" became the ultimate in flexibility for many who did not need the benefits of full-time employment. The irony of this practice is that over time it puts more and more pressure on the permanent full-time staff to work the less-desirable shifts. For one of NAI's client organizations, the net effect was that over a three-year period more and more staff went casual. This continued until a new executive team put a halt to the practice and stabilized the full-time staff complement. Clearly, staffing flexibility and ease of internal transfers are important, but they cannot be introduced without balance. Individual needs should be taken into account whenever possible, but not at the expense of keeping the organization from discharging its ultimate responsibility—the delivery of excellent patient care.

Recognition

During the 1980s, recognition and noncompensation "incentive" programs were quite popular in the manufacturing industry as a way of generating loyalty. Ten years later, they caught on in health-care. Used as a way of saying thanks and to promote institutional loyalty, employees can save points that can be redeemed for merchandise. The practice can also backfire with many employee groups who regard the redemptions as an infantilization of loyalty and an avoidance of dealing with the really important systemic issues that lie at the heart of the problem. Although recognition is important, programmatic or institutional recognition programs do not motivate individual behavior. As we will discuss in Chapter 5, the recognition that is motivating occurs at the level of the individual and one-up manager, not in broad-brush approaches.

Task Forces and Employee Surveys

If done well, employee surveys are critically important sources of data about the organization's health and many yield turnover and labor-relations vulnerability indices. Although the process of doing surveys provides an important message about people management and employee concerns, what's done with the data is the most critical factor. Sadly, many organizations "do employee surveys" but do not have mechanisms in place to ensure that issues that surface are effectively resolved. Asking for opinions and doing nothing about them will undermine morale faster than not asking at all.

Similarly, recruitment and retention task forces are common in many healthcare organizations. They have broad-based task forces at the hospital or organizational level with half that number employing task forces at the system level. But are task forces "retention methods"? As problem identification and resolution groups they may generate solutions (i.e., methods) for dealing with retention, but by themselves they are not methods as the following example illustrates.

In one of the top hospitals in the survey a retention task force was initiated five years ago to deal with what was then an incipient problem—the availability of experienced surgery nurses. The work on the surgery unit had become increasingly difficult, and recruitment efforts weren't securing the best staff. For the same money, nurses could work at other institutions within the region with a lot less perceived stress because of the complexity of their patient population. New surgical techs and new nurses put more pressure on the more experienced staff who were pulled into service by irritated physicians who didn't want their cases staffed by "newbies." Those newcomers who did opt to join the surgery specialty teams went through their orientations in record time. Mostly driven by cost constraints and the need to have bodies staff the operating rooms, the orientations had been shortened from 16 weeks to 2 to 3 weeks.

Because "democratic" rule had taken hold, everyone served as a preceptor to someone. So, not surprisingly, skills were highly inconsistent because preceptors were not constant, were not responsible for providing feedback to their new staff, and were not held accountable for the new staff member's success. Frequently, new staff were interrogated during cases, made to feel as though they were incompetent, and made to understand that they were not ready to take on the work load expected. A case of blaming the victim? Perhaps. Not surprisingly, turnover was very high. Yet the department's recruitment and retention task force, which met on this issue weekly for over 18 months, defined the problem as "inadequacy on the part of newer staff to meet the demands of the work environment." So the turnover revolving door continued to bring in new, well-intended clinical staff who were placed in positions beyond their capabilities to fill the gaps left by experienced staff and recent hires who were leaving through the back door.

Staffing

Unfortunately, only 11 percent of respondents noted that responding to issues of inadequate staffing and extraordinarily large management spans of control were retention methods. Clearly, given the discussion of issues in Chapter 1, staffing and span-of-control issues must be a dominant focus of any serious attempt to solve the problem of retention in healthcare.

PERCEIVED EFFECTIVENESS OF FREQUENTLY USED RETENTION METHODS

Retention Methods Perceived as Most Effective

Survey participants were asked to identify the effectiveness of the retention methods that they used. Table 3.2 identifies those methods that participants believed were the most effective among all the methods they were actually using. Even though a small percentage

Table 3.2: Retention Methods Perceived as Effective

Retention Method	Respondents Who Identified Method as "Most Effective"
Preference to internal promotion	100%
Compensation	62%
Discretionary salary adjustments	57%
Retention bonuses	38%
Retention task force	37%
Upgrade the health plan	36%
Top-management attendance at meetings	36%

of institutions used it (11 percent), "preference to internal promotion" was perceived to have maximum impact by every respondent who employed this approach. This finding is consistent with studies in other industries that indicate lack of advancement opportunities as a major reason for voluntary separations. Offering further support for the importance of internal promotion is the fact that those organizations in the survey that used this method experienced lower turnover than those that didn't.

Compensation interventions, including reviews, salary adjustments, and retention bonuses, were also cited among the most-effective techniques used. How much of this "success" was the result of "keeping up with the Joneses" is an important question, bearing in mind the discussion earlier in this chapter. "Discretionary salary adjustments" were deemed effective in reducing turnover by more than half of the hospitals that employed them. To maximize the effectiveness of this approach, however, managers must have the authority to recognize superior performance based on specific criteria. Otherwise, the process feeds the perception of politically motivated deployment of bonus dollars. The failure to objectively differentiate between adequate and superior performance can be a significant demotivator for employees, regardless of their position or experience. Given the large spans of control, credible performance feedback is rare. Without such feedback, discretionary salary adjustments are likely to be regarded as political.

Retention bonuses, although necessary in keeping up with current market practices, were deemed effective by only 38 percent of respondents. They are clearly a more reactive approach because they implicitly acknowledge the possibility that staff will go elsewhere. Perhaps more importantly, retention bonuses, like signing bonuses, raise the mean salary within the geographical area. As noted earlier, employees tend to transition to different institutions to collect the bonuses!

As described before, a retention task force is a means to arrive at a solution to a problem. It should not be confused with the solution itself. Whether or not a task force serves as an effective way to find solutions depends on a variety of factors such as its makeup, leadership, ability to think out of the box, analytic depth, etc.

Clearly, hospitals need to tailor their benefits, strategy, and structure for the population segments represented in their existing and potential workforce. Many strategies are possible. If you're trying to encourage longer tenure among those who conceivably can retire, you might reconfigure your pension/retirement plan. If, on the other hand, you're focused on new entrants to the workforce, you might provide child care coverage. In short, no one answer is right in all circumstances.

Given the fact that the average age of healthcare workers is increasing, "upgrading the health benefit plan" can encourage employees to remain with their current institution. Although many healthcare workers express serious concern when they learn that they may be ineligible for continued benefits on retirement, those institutions that can provide even prorated benefits may still get a few extra years from them.

"Top-management's attendance at meetings," the last item on the perceived most-effective list, is important for visibility and linking senior managers to the issues and concerns within the organization. As noted earlier, visibility, access, and communication represent good practice. However, such attendance and visibility should not be regarded as retention tools.

Retention Methods Perceived as Least Effective

Table 3.3 lists the retention methods judged least effective by respondents. Three of the five least-effective retention methods are related to employee benefits. Essentially, these benefits were not perceived by respondents as an effective influencer in employees' decisions to stay with the hospital. As noted earlier, "upgrading the health plan" made the top retention tool list as perceived by survey respondents. Yet it appears on the least effective list as well. How do we explain this? If benefits are structured to meet the needs of the employee population base, then they are an important part of the retention mix. However, given distinctly different employee populations, what is attractive to one may have little appeal to another. Thus, tuition reimbursement may be a great recruitment tool for those who plan to go back to school. However, it will create resentment for that cadre of current employees who have been out of school for two to three years and are heavily in debt. In a similar view, focus on retirement is highly relevant for baby boomers and irrelevant for many generation Xers. Given the expense involved in changing benefit plans there are important lessons here. Extensive thought and research should go into decisions regarding benefit changes because once installed they become demotivators if removed, regardless of whether or not they served as motivators in the first place! Not surprisingly then, "upgrading the health plan" appeared on both the most-effective and least-effective lists.

Increasing benefit payouts, like upgrading healthcare plans, is often a reaction to other institutions who have raised the stakes. Although the initial impact can appear significant, the effect is often time limited, as other institutions likewise respond and the novelty wears off.

Table 3.3: Retention Methods Perceived as Least Effective

Retention Method	Respondents Who Identified Methods as "Least Effective"
Employee-issues hotline	67%
Flexible benefits	43%
Upgrade the health plan	36%
Improve the retirement/pension plan	33%
Hospital-branded merchandise	31%

Although two-thirds of respondents listed "employee-issues hotline" as a least-effective method of retention, it continues to be a necessary component in engendering good will among staff. As discussed earlier, the hotline should not be regarded as a method to reduce turnover, but it is effective in providing insight into issues that may themselves lead to turnover if unattended.

"Hospital-branded merchandise," the last item on the list perceived to be ineffective yet frequently used, represents an attempt to forge institutional identification. It attempts to create the conditions that simulate employee bonding and identification. When people choose to wear the name of their employer, it implies personal endorsement. But giving people (or expecting them to buy) hospital-branded merchandise does not in itself create that identification or endorsement. Such extrinsic representations can never be a substitute for the intrinsic motivation that retention requires.

EMPLOYEE SURVEYS AND OTHER RETENTION METHODS

Employee Survey Data

Because 58 percent of the hospitals listed surveys as a retention tool, respondents were also asked about how they actually used employee surveys, even though they didn't appear on either the most-effective or least-effective retention methods lists. Respondents reported that typically, the survey analysis was broken down by department level or less frequently at the unit level within the department. Most of the responsibility for action based on survey results lay with the department manager or at the human resources level. However, committees and focus groups were often used to recommend actions/steps in response to the data. Some of the actions resulting from employee surveys at responding organizations included adjustments in pay, development of retention training programs, and "upgrades" in communication with senior management. Quite surprisingly, few hospitals built in any meaningful accountability for change as a result of survey scores at the unit-manager level, either because the data were not available to evaluate adequacy or impact of management practices at that level or because the process itself did not have teeth. As we'll discuss in Chapter 6, best practices organizations hold managers accountable for the impact of management practices in the same way that managers are held accountable for financial performance.

As illustrated in Figure 3.1, surveys were perceived as most effective by 23 percent of respondents who used them and least effective by 18 percent of those that used them, which is a significant disparity in the perceived utility of surveys as a retention tool. This discrepancy reflects the fact that employee surveys, at their most basic level, provide a vehicle for employee input and interaction by serving as a critical feedback mechanism. They are not by themselves a retention method, in the same way that a speedometer is not a safety device. Surveys can provide management with valuable climate and "satisfaction" data that can be used to predict retention and assess the actual effectiveness of management practices. Unfortunately, most institutions don't use survey data this way. If they did, results could be incorporated into specific managerial objectives for which department managers could be held

Figure 3.1: Perceived Effectiveness of Surveys as a Retention Tool

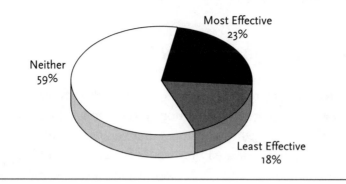

accountable. An example of this objective is "increase (specific) management practice scores from X to Y over the next year."

Another important and legitimate application for surveys is in documenting employee issues, identifying vulnerabilities, and assessing impact of actions taken. Organizations that do this systematically subsequently decrease their turnover. With proper design and a rigorous follow-up process, employee surveys can serve as an enormously effective tool for managing the factors that control retention.

On a related note, we know that direct line managers have the most immediate and visible impact on employee turnover. Because half of the respondents held their department managers accountable for retention, respondents were asked what specific actions their hospital was taking to help first-line managers to be more effective in retaining employees. Almost half of the respondents reported that they were offering more leadership development training to managers to help them "coach" employees and to develop skills that promote retention. Approximately one-third of the respondents said they communicated more information to managers—primarily turnover data and the results of employee surveys. Instituting structured intervention by human resources was another initiative mentioned by a third of the hospitals. This consists of assisting in hiring and exit interviews, providing toolkits to facilitate retention, and putting compensation systems in place, including merit increases, that support retention.

SURVEY RESPONDENTS' PLANS

As noted in Chapter 1, 85 percent of hospitals surveyed reported they were devoting more attention to retention than they had in the past. When asked what future initiatives they would be pursuing, ten hospitals indicated they would be reviewing and "upgrading compensation" (see Table 3.4). Examples of compensation upgrades included pay system revisions to ensure competitiveness, bonuses, and premium and seminar pay. This trend is consistent with perceptions that upgrading compensation is an effective retention tool among those who already use it. However, as discussed earlier in this chapter, such "effectiveness" may be temporary. When upgrading compensation, all hospitals in the market are likely to follow suit to match the competition. This trend results in inflating the standard salary range in that labor market rather than differentiating that hospital as a better-paying employer or an employer of choice for other reasons. The net long-term effect is a higher base compensation level, not loyalty, across all hospitals at a time when hospitals can ill afford the expense.

Attempts to engage employees, and thereby seek loyalty and retention through increased input, included implementing suggestion boxes, having staff serve on committees, and instituting employee surveys. Although each of these methods has merit, caution should be exercised. Input, also known as participation, can engage employees in meaningful ways if structured appropriately. However, as will be discussed in chapters 5 and 7, strategic role clarity and clear performance expectations must be in place for input to be meaningful. Without such elements, energized chaos is the likely result. Moreover, input that receives no response raises expectations that can't or won't be met. The net result is lowered morale and conditions for increased turnover.

Table 3.4: Future Initiatives to Address Retention

Rank	Initiative
1	Upgrade compensation
2	Increase input
3	Identify termination reasons
	Upgrade education/training
4	Improve benefits
5	Improve staffing/scheduling
	Refine turnover tracking and reporting systems

Several respondents noted their commitment to "upgrade education and training." These planned initiatives consist of providing more management and leadership development training and encouraging staff education as an incentive to retention. Assuming these efforts offer an integrated approach to developing management depth and competence, we applaud this direction. Tying development for managers and employees into succession planning and career pathing will go a long way to further retention while improving organizational effectiveness.

One way to contain turnover is to understand its roots and provide targeted responses to the causes. Being able to "identify termination reasons" is an approach that is critical to the successful management of turnover. Systematically conducting exit interviews is the most common and valid means to achieving this, assuming they are structured appropriately and the data are analyzed effectively. One respondent reported that specific issues would be aggregated by job groups and addressed accordingly. Along these same lines, four hospitals reported that they planned to "refine turnover tracking and reporting systems" to provide turnover data by department and disseminate turnover information more broadly. This is a proactive step toward effective measurement and effectively reduces some of the measurement gaps discussed in Chapter 2. Other frequent responses included to "improve benefits" and "improve staffing/scheduling." Although benefits and flexible scheduling were not cited as being particularly effective in addressing turnover, both can be seen as "table stakes" necessary to keep up with industry standards.

CONCLUSION

Twenty-seven (27) different and distinct retention methods, which fall into unique clusters, were identified by survey participants. Not surprisingly, compensation, benefits, and training/development comprised the bulk of methods employed to address retention issues. What's important to know is that although many of these methods were frequently used and believed to be effective, they ultimately were not and some (particularly a number related to compensation and benefits) in fact were even self-defeating. Ironically, the most unanimously perceived effective method—internal promotion—was not widely used and should have been, assuming competencies had been systematically built. On the other hand, at least some hospitals were treating data gathering and analysis as retention tools. Although these are critical tools for understanding the problem of retention, they are not solutions or remedies. Finally, much work still needs to be done to better define compensation and benefits strategies and relate them to the hospital's individual competitive situation and brand.

CHAPTER 4

Communication Mechanisms for Employee Involvement

THE LATE DON JACKSON, a psychiatrist interested in the problems of communication, is credited for noting that one cannot not communicate. As you journey through this chapter, the significance of this truism will become increasingly apparent. Our findings emphasize that communication is one of management's most important activities, one that is deceptively simple and surprisingly complex at the same time.

The complexity of communication is quickly brought to light in the following example, which reflects experiential aspects of management training seminars we have led over the years. The experiment began with a trainee who volunteered to lead her colleagues in a task. She was presented with a 4x6 index card on which was drawn the geometric design in Figure 4.1. The group was told to draw the figure, following her instructions. However, no one could ask any questions in executing her drawings, and she was to instruct them with her back to the group! This way she could not respond to any difficulties the group might be having because she had no way of knowing what they were. This was designed as a no-feedback environment. After completing the drawing, the group was asked to begin the experiment again. This

Figure 4.1: Geometric Design Experiment

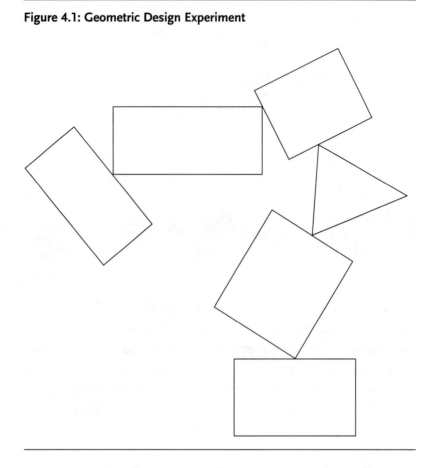

time the volunteer faced the group as she gave instructions. Group members asked questions, and she could even give specific recommendations to them to improve their drawing accuracy. This was a feedback environment.

Results of this training "experiment" were quite interesting. Almost twice as much time was required to complete the task in the second environment as compared to the first. Participants' accuracy in replicating the drawing in the second environment was markedly improved compared to their accuracy in the first, no-feedback environment. Their frustration in the first environment was quite high, and their level of involvement in the task actually decreased as the task progressed. The opposite was true in the second environment where involvement increased and frustration was minimal. However, the leader's own feeling of self-confidence in her ability to communicate was higher in the first environment. In addition, she expected participants' drawings to be executed accurately. She was quite surprised to learn that they were not accurate and tended to "blame" the participants for not following directions!

What lessons can be learned from this experiment?

1. Feedback seems to make a real difference in the accuracy of performance.
2. Feedback takes more time.
3. Participants (e.g., employees) who do not have the opportunity for feedback and dialog (e.g., asking questions regarding performance and task exceptions, clarifying direction, and so on) may experience unnecessary frustration and feel uninvolved in the task.
4. Leaders (e.g., managers and executives) may have an unwarranted sense of self-confidence and believe that their expectations and directions have been communicated clearly and received when, in fact, they have not been.
5. When leaders operate from such a position, they are likely to believe that performance errors are the result of participants' or employees' inadequacies, not of interpersonal-communication difficulties in which they share 50 percent of the responsibility.
6. Participants ask for clarification on a particular point in terms of their own frame of reference. This means that the same question will be asked in several different ways.

This example represents an artificial situation, but its relevance should not be lost. All the participants were executives, managers, or supervisors in healthcare organizations. At the time, they were all easily able to relate this experience to life in the real world. For instance, first-line supervisors and managers are frequently pressed for time. As a result, they give directions to employees quickly, without soliciting or encouraging feedback to ascertain that the intent of what they have communicated has been received. When employees go off to perform the task in question and perform inadequately, supervisors frequently become irritated, often criticizing their employees for not following directions. Having been criticized makes it likely that these employees won't ask for feedback the next time around.

In short, communication is the tool through which we discover the world around us and our relationship to it. Given that communication is the vehicle for exchanging meaning and learning about others' expectations, intentions, and their reactions to us, etc., it is really the bridge between people. It is the means through which people get involved, get validated, and get close to each other and the organization that employs them. Because of this, understanding communication as a mechanism for employee involvement is essential to understanding the complex mechanism of retention and why retention is not just about benefits and compensation.

Good communication, whether one way or two way, is generally considered to be positively correlated with better retention results. However, not all communication mechanisms are created equal or have comparable results. Some communication media, such as organizational surveys, are clearly more effective than others in a healthcare environment. Understanding what makes a medium more or less effective sets the stage for our discussion of what the top-100 hospitals in our survey used to communicate.

This chapter examines the survey results on this topic, graphically representing the communication mechanisms for employee involvement most frequently employed by respondents. We also make recommendations based on our experience in working with organizations that effectively build employee loyalty and improve retention outcomes.

SETTING THE CONTEXT: UNDERSTANDING THE DRIVERS OF EFFECTIVE COMMUNICATION

Communication involves the exchange of information between two individuals, between an individual and a group, or between groups. In an organizational setting, the complexity of this information exchange and the need to craft messages carefully for different audiences is often underestimated. Frequently, the message that's received is very different from the one that's intended. The extent to which messages are received as intended depends on a number of factors such as shared values, common experience, clarity of the message, appropriateness of the communication vehicle, level of trust, openness to new ideas, etc. What determines effectiveness is the clarity of what's communicated to a given audience, how it's communicated, and the vehicle through which it's communicated. In addition, expectations of outcomes from the communication must be aligned. If any of these elements are missing or weak, then communication is likely to be impaired.

There are a variety of ways in which information exchanges take place. For simplicity sake, we can categorize them along two dimensions: (1) the extent of interaction (real time, time-shifted, or no interaction) and (2) the origin (bottom up, top down, mutual), as seen in Figure 4.2. Based on the model, management may communicate from the top down with or without time-shifted dialog. For example, the hospital's web site, newsletter, and letters from the CEO are examples of top-down communication without dialog. What's important in this model is that neither the sender nor the receiver expect dialog, so when it doesn't happen expectations are not misaligned.

Quarterly management forums and all associate meetings are examples of top-down, real-time communication, where the expectation is that big-picture information (e.g., the state of the organization) will be offered with some limited opportunity for question and answer. The latter represents acceptable real-time

Figure 4.2: Communication Modalities, by Type

		No Interaction	Real Time	Time Shifted
Origin	Top Down	• Newsletters • Web sites • Letters from CEO	• Quarterly management meetings • Annual administration updates	• E-mails
	Mutual	N/A	• Townhall meetings • Staff meetings • Committees, task forces • CEO breakfasts	N/A
	Bottom Up	• Exit interviews • Anonymous comments • Employee surveys	• Management access at staff meetings	• E-mails • Suggestion boxes • Hotlines • Employee surveys • Focus groups

Extent of Interaction

communication in this context. On the other hand, e-mail represents top-down, time-shifted communication where the understanding is that exchange is possible but over an extended period of time—that is, time-shifted.

Exit interviews, anonymous comments, and some elements of employee surveys represent bottom-up, no-interaction vehicles. Although these provide important data points from which trends can be discerned, they do not come with any expectation of subsequent feedback or dialog. However, management access at staff meetings provides real-time, bottom-up engagement with senior management. A significant number of bottom-up, time-shifted mechanisms are used in hospitals, including e-mail, suggestion boxes, hotlines, some types of employees surveys, and focus groups. In each of these, input is provided by employees to senior management. Although a response is typically expected at some point in time, there is no expectation that it will be immediate—hence, the label "time shifted."

Finally, mutual real-time communication modalities include town hall and staff meetings, committees, task forces, and CEO breakfasts. In each of these, there is an expectation that communication exchange will, in fact, be mutual—that is, that a dialog will occur. To the extent such expectations are not met, frustration is likely for initial offenses. Over a period of time, misaligned expectations can lead to withdrawal and cynicism.

HIGHLIGHTING THE FREQUENTLY USED COMMUNICATION METHODS

What does the foregoing discussion mean for communication in hospitals and the relative effectiveness of various modalities?

Because communication, access, and visibility are critical to retention and building loyalty, survey respondents were asked how their hospitals communicate with and solicit input from staff. Table 4.1 describes the most frequently used methods for communication and involvement. Each of these will be discussed separately.

Meetings

By far, the most popular venue across all types of organizations was "meetings." This category included regularly scheduled staff meetings and special forums and town halls. Based on the discussion and models presented earlier in the chapter, meetings clearly represent the opportunity for real-time dialog and thus have the potential to create the greatest connection between employees and management. Although meetings were the most popular venues noted by respondents for communicating, the method was only used by 32 percent. In addition, the nature of large-scale forums and town halls (included in this category) makes intimate connection impossible merely

Table 4.1: Most Frequently Used Communication and Involvement Methods

Rank	Respondents Who Used the Method	Method
1	32%	Meetings (e.g, staff, quarterly, administration, town hall)
2	31%	Newsletters (e.g., general, department, position, issue)
3	24%	Committees (e.g., communications, nursing, task forces)
3	24%	E-communication (e.g., web site, electronic bulletin board services)
5	18%	Management access (e.g., attendance at staff meetings)
6	11%	Focus groups (e.g., communication, customer service)
7	8%	Enhanced management communication
8	5%	Hotlines, suggestion boxes, exit interviews
9	4%	Other (e.g., internal communication, quality assurance process, and shared governance)

because of their size. Although these are excellent vehicles for dialog if structured well, many have become a platform for broadcast communications from senior management to an uncomfortable audience. The latter group is likely to engage in post-meeting meetings to discuss its real reactions to the material presented because the venue doesn't allow for open, two-way discussion of any depth.

In contrast are staff meetings that, when structured effectively, become an excellent vehicle for dialog, setting context, clarifying expectations, talking through issues, and building the work team. Staff meetings, in particular, are critical to connecting people to the organization through their immediate manager. In recent years, unfortunately, many organizations have eliminated these types of meetings as part of their expense-control measures. The rationale was clear: anything not directly associated with direct care was expendable. People have frequently been asked to spend their own time, not reimbursed, in some organizations to attend staff meetings. The assumption is that professional staff will value staff meetings. When they didn't volunteer their time, no direct consequences ensued. Meetings just stopped and with them management's ability to connect with the group. Such decisions have weakened ties between employees and management and have contributed to such consequences as increased turnover. When staff meetings are conducted, polls of employees suggest that many are regarded as a waste of time. Our contention is that this view holds because most meetings are poorly structured.

The Case for Reinstating Regular and Well-Planned Staff Meetings

It is important to conduct meetings on a regular basis because they provide a sense of continuing structure for employees. Such meetings provide a consistent venue during which individuals know they can count on receiving information and/or expressing their views. In smaller departmental or unit meetings, staff members also have an opportunity to connect with members of their own team, which provides a higher comfort level for interaction and feedback. Clearly the level of interaction varies across groups, in part depending on the number of individuals participating in the meeting. Typically the smaller the number of individuals involved, the higher the level of free-flowing exchange of ideas. This may not always be appropriate, of course, particularly when meetings are held strictly for the purpose of conveying information and answering specific questions such as what might occur at an introduction of new insurance benefits. However, in departmental or unit settings, well-structured and well-led meetings can take the form of problem solving and exchange sessions.

Such sessions carry with them a very clear and powerful message: management values staff ideas and opinions. Thus, meetings can increase employee identification and buy in, but only if they are well designed and structured.

There are standard guidelines that should be followed in conducting meetings. For example, an agenda should always be used to guide the flow of information and discussion. This organizing principle enables participants to anticipate upcoming topics. The best planned meetings help those in attendance prepare for discussion. Prework and a limited number of "thought" questions, which will be used to guide the discussion, are most helpful in generating rich meetings. Tools, such as meeting minutes, that serve as a reminder later about what was discussed are also critical. It is always helpful to record and distribute meeting minutes. The minutes provide documentation of what transpired during the meeting and ensure that everyone involved is on the same page whether or not they attended. Minutes are also required by funding organizations and accrediting bodies to prove that the meeting occurred, to reflect actions taken during the meeting, and to reflect assignments after the meeting.

Newsletters

"Newsletters," cited by 31 percent of respondents as a communication or involvement technique, may be produced in various forms and require a great deal of energy if they're going to be done well. Newsletters are an example of top-down, one-way communication (i.e., without interaction). They are a static vehicle and thus share the pitfalls of the no-feedback environment described at the beginning of this chapter. However, as part of the communication mix they serve an important role. As an adjunct to well-structured meetings they can clearly crystallize key points that then get distributed to a wide audience. Although people will read between the lines to see what messages are intended, newsletters can represent the facts in a consistent, nonemotional but engaging way, which is particularly useful in controversial situations. They represent the tangibles discussed in the meeting, providing a history of important items.

They are most effective as a way to directly represent the voice of senior leadership or nursing administration, whose day-to-day exposure to the broader employee base is limited. Directors and managers can then be positioned as being on the same page in this context by being quoted and by giving local examples to illustrate points. Newsletters may be structured as regular organizationwide publications distributed monthly or quarterly, or they may be structured by department or position such as a nursing newsletter. Sometimes, newsletters focus on an issue such as providing explanations for large-scale organizational changes; these newsletters are often stuffed in paycheck envelopes to facilitate the likelihood of being read.

When a question-and-answer section is included, the newsletter simulates some aspects of time-shifted communication and thus provides more engagement power, assuming the information is seen as credible. Employee accomplishments can also provide positive content for newsletters, although it is important to ensure broad departmental exposure across the hospital. If nursing's accomplishments are the only ones noted in an organizationwide newsletter on a consistent basis, the credibility of the publication will diminish with staff in other areas. By publicizing employee accomplishments, the values of the organization can be promoted highlighting individuals and groups who stand for important aspects of the culture.

Committees

"Committees," cited by 24 percent of respondents, may provide two-way communication, depending on their composition and proper implementation. Thus, committees have the potential to serve as mutual, real-time communication vehicles. This category included committees for specific departments or functions (such as nursing committees) or for particular purposes (such as task forces). A retention task force, referred to in Chapter 3, falls into this category. Although it was beyond the scope of the top-100 hospitals survey to assess the effectiveness of the committees used, our experience in the industry provides important perspectives here.

Although committees play a necessary and vital role in healthcare, a cautionary note on the overuse of committees must be stated. A common complaint by staff members is that they are unable to get enough work accomplished because of an inordinate amount of time they spend in committee meetings. Both standing and ad hoc committees are used extensively in hospital settings, where they are formed to address a multitude of issues. The culture in healthcare settings has supported this form of problem solving for a number of years. Part of the reason for the bias toward forming committees is that many committees are actually required by payers and accrediting agencies such as the Joint Commission on Accreditation of Healthcare Organizations. Beyond this, a committee orientation is supported by the social interaction available at committee meetings, the social value associated with being part of an exclusive group, and a nursing culture that eschews individual leadership in favor of participative decision making. Some organizations have actually made committee participation, not effectiveness, a criterion for performance appraisal. Such policies effectively penalize those staff members who insist on allocating their time in ways they believe will yield more significant outcomes. In many institutions, such factors have led to a proliferation of committees that, without "sunshine" rules, convene indefinitely and that, without adequate structure or accountability for results, often tend to consume far more resources than they can justify by their output.

Given that committees are a necessary part of the landscape, how can they be structured and managed to achieve optimal efficiency? First, committees must be chartered with a very clear purpose, and appropriate membership must be selected. The organization also needs to define the reasonable estimated life of the group and communicate this to the committee chair along with reporting time frames and acceptable deliverables. Many committee structures within and outside the industry lack clear charters or purpose. Such lack of clarity sets the group on an inefficient if not ineffective journey. Without clarity, membership selection is more likely to become politicized and expand in ways that jeopardize outcomes.

Once the purpose of a committee is clear, creating a core team of topical experts becomes possible. Clearly, these experts must represent their colleagues, and they can also bring breadth of perspectives. The core team's efforts can be supplemented by ad hoc or sub task groups to work on more narrowly defined issues under the general direction of the specific general committee. Time frames provide the necessary focus and structure to move the work along at a reasonable pace. Without time frames, "scope creep" takes over and committees wind up having a life of their own. Providing such structure prevents the problem of retention task forces that go on discussing issues for months without bringing viable solutions.

E-Communication

"E-communication," mentioned by 24 percent of respondents, can also be two way but is rarely interactive and is not as heavily used in healthcare as it is in other industries. It is characterized as a top-down or bottom-up time-shifted modality in Figure 4.2.

The most predominant form of e-communication is e-mail. This can be an efficient use of time, creating the opportunity to compose and disseminate information quickly and effectively to multiple persons. Another benefit is that fewer resources, such as paper, toner, and the internal mailing system, are used than in distributing a standard memo. Further, e-mail saves time in conveying information compared to placing a phone call, which can result in an extended conversation. If not used properly, however, e-mail can actually add time.

It must be recognized that e-mail can become problematic when used extensively in place of face-to-face contact. In addition, e-mail provides easy access to anyone within an organization and may become overused for broadcast messages, thereby overwhelming recipients in terms of sheer volume. If this becomes a significant communication device, appropriate limits must be placed on using e-mail in lieu of personal contact. For example, e-mail distribution lists should be scrutinized so that only those individuals who are affected by the content or have legitimate need for knowing the content are included. Although no data exist that define the number of e-mails that can be productively passed between people, the rule of common sense should prevail. Perhaps most importantly, topics that are likely to be controversial should be introduced in person and worked through in real time.

Other types of e-communication are electronic bulletin boards and web sites. Web sites are a good source of internal information, including job openings and other news. The problem with relying on a web site to disseminate information is that there is no guarantee that employees will take the time to access the site and receive information. Electronic bulletin boards allow employees to post comments and questions and review other employee discussions online. These provide a rich resource for discussion on policies and procedures and information on clinical applications and new equipment. Bulletin boards should be monitored, however, to ensure that incorrect information is not being disseminated and used, resulting in serious medical consequences.

E-communication is also used to provide broadcasts of events, such as recognition lunches, on the hospital intranet system. Employees can actually watch from their own computer an awards ceremony as it occurs at a remote location. The same principle holds true for speakers and surgical procedures, where employees have the opportunity to view the engagement without actually being there.

Two factors associated with e-communication should be pointed out. First, management needs to ensure that employees don't spend an excessive amount of time on e-communication activities. Staff may find it more entertaining to "play" on the computer than to perform assigned responsibilities. "Surfing the net" has become a national pastime, and managers need to monitor time spent on recreational activities rather than job-related duties. In most cases, people don't abuse this situation; however, it is still a factor to be considered. Second, in many hospitals, nonmanagement employees don't readily have access to computer terminals. Terminals may be shared among a number of people or located in managers' offices. This certainly limits the functionality of e-communication as well as creates privacy issues. However, this is the reality of the situation.

Management Access

"Management access," reported by 18 percent of respondents, involves top-management attendance at staff meetings, meals with the CEO, birthday celebrations, etc. Although this provides the presence of senior management, it does not guarantee an exchange of communication. Generally, employees appreciate the opportunity to spend time with top management and to express their views. It is critical that during these times the CEO or other top-management member make a concerted effort to actively interact with staff and to remain open and nonjudgmental. Otherwise, the meeting will be seen as an exercise in insincere public relations, where employees must be asked to restrain themselves to ensure they "don't rock the boat" and thus face consequences. It is usually effective to invite staff to volunteer to serve as representatives at meetings with the CEO. Small group (15 to 20 participants) venues facilitate more open exchange, and even with a small group there's likely to be more impact by randomizing participation to reduce duplication among the attendees.

Another method for achieving management access is to have CEOs and other top managers increase their visibility within the organization, whether that means walking the halls or eating in the employee lunchroom. Our experience has shown that employees are more positive about an organization when they have seen top executives walking around rather than isolating themselves in executive offices. Staff members want to be able to put a face with the name of their leader, not just when the leader is at the podium during a meeting but also out in the "field." This instills greater employee confidence in the leader's ability to relate to employee issues. Another benefit of being visible in the halls is that CEOs and top executives can interface with patients and their families, keeping in touch with their customers. The challenge here is for executives to be familiar enough that their presence is comfortable and not disruptive to employees. If they are uncomfortable with the venue, their comments are likely to be seen as insincere. Their insincerity will undermine any value such management access is likely to bring. For executives who are uncomfortable with informal settings, it's more effective to create more structured question-and-answer sessions, even if the questions are submitted in advance and the answers are prepared.

One CFO at one of the top-100 hospitals in the survey learned this lesson the hard way. In an attempt to become more accessible he toured his facility with the chief nursing officer (CNO). As they entered one of the critical care units, he innocently asked an RN, "How is it going?" She curtly replied, "It's not going well, and if you can't help with patients then I don't have time to talk." The CNO then explained that this was the reality of operating short staffed, which she had tried to get him to understand for a year in meeting after meeting. This experience left an indelible mark on the CFO, but it didn't improve his image among the staff. Clearly this is not the norm, and there are many examples of excellent access and visibility described in

Chapter 6. But it does highlight the need for ongoing and real management access.

Focus Groups

"Focus groups" were used by 11 percent of the respondents as an input mechanism. They represent a bottom-up, time-shifted modality as depicted in Figure 4.2. Originally used as a type of market-research tool, focus groups typically involve a small number of people (8 to 12) asked to participate because they have a viewpoint on the subject at hand that management wants to hear. Focus group participants are encouraged by a facilitator to engage in open dialog around a particular issue or set of questions. The advantage of a focus group, in contrast to a survey, is that richer information can be gleaned—that is, if the venue is structured well. Participants may be asked their opinions on a series of questions, to respond to a scenario, or to engage in brainstorming around an issue. Because it is meant to allow people to speak in relatively free form around specific topics, a focus group may be used to elicit issues from which a detailed survey will be designed that can then yield quantitative results with large groups. The focus group may also be used post survey to help flesh out solutions to issues identified through the survey. Regardless of how they are used, they may be issue specific or of a general nature such as improving employee morale.

When using focus groups, it is important to carefully determine the composition. Different individuals should be used representing diverse areas of the organization so as not to bias the results toward one group. Conducting multiple focus groups may be helpful, with each group representing a specific segment of the organization to elicit greater depth from departmental perspectives. Often, in a mixed group, participants are not forthcoming with information that they perceive is unpopular with the group. In a focus group comprising like-minded individuals, such as all administrative support or all environmental services staff, participants are more likely to be open and vocal with their opinions.

By summarizing information by group and then comparing results across groups, rich trends can be seen that may not become clear if strongly felt views are not expressed because of discomfort in the group. For this reason some focus groups made up of heterogeneous members are structured using a nominal group process technique. Essentially this technique enables each participant to jot down his or her thoughts on the issue privately. The facilitator goes around the room eliciting an idea from each participant until all ideas are captured. Discussion then ensues. In this way, all ideas, no matter how controversial, are laid out. For this process to work well, the facilitator must be an expert in managing group process.

Even though participants in the top-100 hospital survey spontaneously listed focus groups as a communication/involvement vehicle, it should be noted that this is a modality targeted to receiving structured input. What is critical in managing the modality effectively is for management to summarize the inputs and provide feedback to participants and a broader audience on what has or will be done with the insights gleaned. Although they are a time-shifted medium, focus groups bring an expectation that the feedback loop will be closed. Failure to do so will undermine management's credibility and put a wedge between the organization and its workforce.

Enhancing Management Communication

For communication to be effective it must engage participants in a dialog. Unfortunately, a great deal of communication across industries reflects the broadcast-and-review variety and leaves the dialog to the grapevine and the hallway. Particularly in healthcare organizations, this approach translates frequently to a read-and-initial philosophy. This philosophy, in turn, reflects the reality of 24/7 operations and the logistical challenge for managers. How can they touch all of their staff members who work selected shifts across the entire week?

Without the supporting infrastructure, "read and initial" becomes the only available method of communicating nonemergent information. Unfortunately, this method is passive. It leaves out context and strategic understanding and lets in assumptions. Without the opportunity to engage in meaningful dialog about the substance, intent, and implications of the policy, memo, etc., no real commitment; buy-in; and, ultimately, compliance are possible. Even when meetings are held, they often wind up resembling oral versions of read and initial. This occurs largely because administration assumes that managers and supervisors know how to plan and structure an effective meeting and, once there, have mastered the art of effective meeting facilitation and group problem solving. Unfortunately, mastering the real power of structured communication, dialog, and effective meeting management is not a generally held competency.

The importance of managerial communication was cited by 8 percent of respondents. The fact that only 8 percent of respondents offered this as an example of a vehicle they used to enhance communication with employees or to provide more opportunities for employee input is a telling statement. Consistent with our commentary in Chapter 1, this result provides additional perspective to the fact that most hospitals do not understand the value of and need for a management infrastructure that engages employees systematically with their immediate managers. When this vehicle was mentioned by survey respondents, the category included communication assistance for managers in the form of talking points for specific topics to ensure that consistent information is communicated throughout the organization. Other organizations offered management training and development on communicating with employees under this category.

Clearly the criticality of communicating with employees across a whole host of subjects—that is, listening to their concerns and responding to them—cannot be underestimated, and neither can the critical role all levels of management must play in making this happen and speaking with one voice.

Hotlines, Suggestion Boxes, and Exit Interviews

Bottom-up communication, from staff to management and administration, consists of employee hotlines, suggestion boxes, and exit interviews. "Employee hotlines," identified by 5 percent of respondents, were discussed in Chapter 3 as a necessary outlet for communication that can serve as a valuable resource in identifying issues. Hotlines allow employees to provide input to top management, either through human resources or CEOs, on an anonymous basis. Hotlines surface important issues and can serve as an outlet for grievances. As discussed in Chapter 3, it is important for managers to follow up on these comments. The same principles hold true for "suggestion boxes."

Although "exit interviews" were only cited by one respondent as a vehicle for input, our experience has shown that they are used extensively throughout healthcare organizations. Typically, an exit interview is perceived as an administrative procedure, mandated by the hospital or regulatory agencies, and viewed as another component of administrative red tape. However, this belief diminishes the potential value of exit interviews. They can be a powerful tool to capture information that is not normally forthcoming in day-to-day operations. Employees who are reluctant to honestly give their opinions while employed for an organization are typically much more willing to be frank as they leave. Departing employees want to speak their mind to clarify their reason for leaving or to improve practices or situations for the remaining employees. Departing employees may view the exit interview as a final service that they can perform for the organization. This practice typically occurs through an interview with the human resource department, which serves as an independent, unbiased audience. Of course, exit interviews are only helpful if results are compiled, trends are identified, and issues are acted on.

These categories—employee hotlines, suggestion boxes, and exit interviews—typically result in one-way communication and bypass immediate supervisors and managers, omitting them from the loop. Surveys are also bottom-up, one-way communication and will be discussed in depth later in this chapter.

Other Methods

Infrequently mentioned modalities for enhancing communication efforts with employees and structuring opportunities for employee input included establishing a communication staff position, the question-and-answer process, and shared governance. Although many hospitals "established communication roles" in the wake of external marketing programs in the late 1980s in particular, many of the internally focused positions were victims of the downsizing and cost cutting that washed over the industry a decade later. It is noteworthy that a couple of institutions are renewing their commitment to internal communications specifically as a mechanism for addressing recruitment and retention issues. Of course, some of the larger facilities never abandoned this important focus.

"Question and answer," as a regulatory requirement, is built into the policies and procedures of all institutions. Positioning this as a vehicle for communication and involvement is unusual, but results can be highly effective if it is done well. To the extent that poor quality is a source of stress and frustration for staff, and thus a contributor to turnover as described in chapters 1 and 5, actively engaging staff in meaningfully improving quality should have a positive impact on retention. The key is in the development of an infrastructure that supports quality improvement, as we will explore in Chapter 5.

But what about "shared governance" as a mechanism for communication and involvement? As discussed in Chapter 1, shared governance began specifically as a structured approach to enhance collaboration between management and nursing staff, with an eye toward increasing involvement of nurses with physicians. As a reaction against the rigid hierarchies seen in many nursing divisions in hospitals around the country, shared governance broke down barriers to communication. However, as we discussed earlier, it also has brought the unfortunate unintended consequence of further undermining the value and subsequent development of a responsive and effective management structure. At its extreme, it has occasionally been the organizationally sanctioned breeding ground for union activity. As one CEO of a major health system remarked:,

> Eighteen months ago, I was very uncomfortable with the energy around shared governance. It seemed to be focused on creating a parallel organization that is separate from the management team. My nursing team looked at the positive side and put enough pressure on me that I agreed to their self-managed experiment. We're paying dearly for that now. By a thin margin, the RN staff voted in the union. At the center (of the activity) was shared governance and the advocates of self-management.

Although it is beyond the scope of this book to discuss in depth the history and impact of shared governance, either as a philosophy or approach to management, it must be understood in the broader context of management. To the extent that it actively engages management with employees in ways that further the organization's mission, purpose, and goals, shared governance's impact is likely to be positive. However, to the extent it undermines the value and integrity of management, its impact will be negative.

THE ROLE OF SURVEYS AS A COMMUNICATION METHOD

Despite the fact that employee surveys were listed by 58 percent of respondents as part of their efforts to deal with retention, none of them identified surveys specifically as a communication tool.

Given that we believe surveys are a critical tool in the communications mix we have chosen to discuss them here.

"Surveys" were listed as most effective by 23 percent of respondents that used them and least effective by 18 percent of those that used them. This represents a significant disparity in the perceived utility of surveys as a retention tool. Despite this variability, it should be recalled (as noted in Chapter 1) that a survey is a critical data-gathering instrument. Depending on how it is used, a survey can produce insights that can dramatically affect turnover rates. Depending on how it is developed, and the database behind it, a survey can highlight areas of vulnerability that can lead to turnover. However, at the most basic level, employee surveys provide a vehicle for employee interaction by serving as a feedback mechanism to management about the impact of management and organization practices. In addition, surveys can serve as a valuable management tool by providing benchmark satisfaction data that, in addition to serving as a predictor of retention, also assess the effectiveness of management practices and associated trends. Results can then be incorporated into managerial objectives. An example management objective can be "to increase strategic role clarity scores from X to Y over the next year." Another application for surveys is in documenting organizationwide employee issues and identifying vulnerabilities that, once addressed, will subsequently result in decreased turnover. With proper design and follow up, employee surveys can serve as an enormously effective tool.

Hospitals that listed surveys as a retention tool were also asked about how they used them. Respondents reported that typically the survey analysis was broken down by department or by unit within the department. Most of the responsibility for acting on survey results fell on the manager or human resources. However, committees and focus groups were often used to recommend broad actions as a result of survey data. Some of the more common recommendations by respondents included adjustments in pay, development of retention training programs, and "upgrades" in communication (e.g., frequency and type of communication).

Although respondents in this study did not report frequency of survey administration and type of questions asked, timing and frequency of survey administration is one of many complex issues connected with this communication intervention and is explored next.

Survey Frequency

For some healthcare organizations, an employee survey is a project run by human resources that is usually put off "until things calm down." Unfortunately, things in healthcare generally seem never to calm down. Waiting for a protracted period of time when no benefits or significant policy changes or no layoffs or dramatic shortages will occur in the hospital or the market area is likely to be a futile undertaking. An employee survey should be administered on a regular schedule, preferably around the same time of year, and its timing should not be dependent on when it's convenient or when employees are more likely to be more positively disposed.

To maximize the value of survey data, employee surveys should be administered every 12 to 24 months. One reason for this is to be able to gauge the impact of organizational responses on survey data. When the hospital acts on survey data by changing policies or initiating communication around an issue, this is when it is useful to readminister the survey so that changes in the data can reasonably be attributed to action that has just been taken. The greater the length of time that elapses between survey administrations, the larger the number of uncontrolled factors that will affect the data. For example, turnover itself guarantees that a readministration will include a number of new employees who bring their own expectations and history to their responses. More time and more extraneous factors can obscure the positive results of organizational response.

On the other hand, there are problems with administering surveys too frequently. One of the most serious concerns involves the issue of "survey fatigue." When patient satisfaction surveys are administered monthly, they are given each time to a new group of patients. These patients only experience the survey once, filling it out based on their most recent hospital stay. In contrast, employees who participate in a survey on a frequent basis complete the same survey repeatedly within the same year. One predictable result of such frequent administration is fatigue with the activity, leading to a lower response rate. This smaller set of respondents is composed of those employees most likely to be motivated to register their opinions—typically those with the most complaints and those who are content to complete the survey with the least amount of thought and effort, which leads to negatively biased and/or less valid data. In addition to the biased sample that artificially depresses scores, the reduced number of respondents means that attempts to look at data from different areas or departments are less valid because the sample is so small.

Another concern with frequent administration is that it does not allow the organization time to act on results and to implement necessary fixes. In addition, it also raises the respondents' awareness of and possible dissatisfaction with issues and expectations for the outcome. Such frequent assessment is like trying to measure a growing child's height with a tape measure every hour. Monthly fluctuations are more likely to represent measurement error in a child's height rather than real change. The same principle holds true with survey administration.

Frequent data collection also raises issues with management of expectations. Our own work and others' studies have found that the act of measuring organizational practices creates expectations in respondents that the resulting data will be acted on (Cammann, Lawler, and Nadler 1980). Surveying employees frequently raises their awareness of issues and dissatisfactions as well as their expectations that improvements will be made. On the practical side, implementing change based on survey results may take some time. This delay will continue to be reflected negatively in results until change comes to fruition. In the process, the survey can become a demotivator for employees who feel that nothing is happening with the results. It can also breed cynicism toward senior management—that is, unless expectations for what is a reasonable response time are actively being managed.

The question, then, becomes what is the optimal frequency for employee surveys? Again, this varies based on size and complexity of the organization. However, our experience has shown that annual implementation is the best barometer of staff satisfaction, allowing enough time to implement changes based on results. In larger organizations, it is more practical to conduct a systemwide survey on a bi-annual basis and then to conduct surveys for a sample of employees on an annual basis. This achieves the balance of getting critical feedback on a timely basis and enables enhancements to take effect and be measured appropriately.

Survey Content

Survey content should be selected carefully to ensure that it will provide the feedback most critical to the organization. Employee surveys should comprise both questions related to the organizational culture and questions related to management practices. This latter category has the most impact on employee retention, as discussed in Chapter 2. The propensity of an individual to stay with an organization is most dependent on his or her interactions with his or her manager, because this is the person with whom daily contact most frequently occurs. Crucial management practices include those related to providing clear expectations for job responsibilities, providing context and accountability for individual contribution to organizational goals, expecting stretch performance goals, engaging in appropriate feedback mechanisms to ensure optimum performance from individuals, and providing a climate where staff members are encouraged to disagree constructively.

Organizational structure elements that should be examined include appropriate spans of control, processes that support the infrastructure (which is addressed in Chapter 5), the standards of excellence that make the organization the "employer of choice" within the community, and career-development opportunities for individuals within the organization. The last element is consistent with the most-effective retention method cited by respondents—that is, having a preference to internal promotion. In both organizational and managerial categories, numerous other elements should be examined on a consistent basis, depending on current issues and hot topics of interest to a particular employer.

Communicating the Results

Once survey data are analyzed, the most critical component of the process is communicating the results. In each organization, there should be a structured plan to ensure that results are disseminated to appropriate constituents and in a uniform way. The worst-case scenario is to have different interpretations of data surfacing throughout the organization. This encourages individuals to form their own conclusions, which may be contrary to actual results. The process for communicating the results should take into account the level of employee or audience. Those in management positions should have detailed results for their area of control, with a feedback process defined that allows them to make sense of the data, communicate results to their staff, and develop action plans with staff input. And they should be held accountable for implementing such plans and improving their practice.

It is important to provide each audience—employees and other stakeholders such as the board of directors—an overview and synopsis geared to each audience's specific concerns and role in the organization. If results, and some information about follow-up plans, are not shared with employees, it will lessen the value of the survey, resulting in a lower response rate in subsequent administrations. If staff members don't feel their input is important and used, they will stop participating in the survey process and begin disengaging from the organization itself. Conducting a survey results in an implicit if not explicit expectation that something will be done with the data. Burying or ignoring the data carries a very powerful and negative message: We're not really interested in hearing your concerns. Conversely, a major benefit of sharing findings and action plans based on results is that employees will feel their contribution to the survey is valued. Together with improved management practices, such value is associated with higher identification with the organization, which is proven to result in higher retention rates.

CONCLUSION

Although responding hospitals generally recognized the importance of communication in managing retention, they failed to recognize that different methods have different effects. The most powerful communication methods—namely those that facilitate meaningful dialog between managers and their staff such as staff meetings—were underutilized. Instead, they relied on broadcast, large-audience methods that provided little interaction. Clearly, these broader-based vehicles reach a larger audience, but they sacrifice effectiveness at the same time. When employee expectations for input and involvement aren't met or hospital administrators do not respond to the concerns they allow to be aired, it sets the stage for cynicism and withdrawal and ultimately turnover. Only by coupling broadcast vehicles with a well-developed management infrastructure will the messages have the desired impact. The components of that infrastructure are the subject of the next chapter.

REFERENCE

Cammann, C., E. E. Lawler III, and D. A. Nadler. 1980. "Perspectives on the Measurement of Organizational Behavior and the Quality of Work Life." In *Organizational Assessment*, pp. 513–14. New York: John Wiley & Sons, Inc.

CHAPTER 5

Building the Infrastructure to Attract and Retain Tomorrow's Workforce

ALTHOUGH TURNOVER MEASUREMENT systems must be put in place, accountability established, retention methods initiated, appropriate cultural norms established, and communication vehicles implemented, long-term success requires that organizations build the infrastructure to support these critical components. This chapter will discuss the specific changes that need to occur to improve retention results as well as ways to structure these changes to ensure success. Through an examination of the basic fundamental functions and processes of healthcare delivery, targeted priority interventions will become clear.

WHAT IS INFRASTRUCTURE?

What exactly do we mean by infrastructure? Essentially, infrastructure refers to the processes, systems, and platforms on which a business runs. Although infrastructure in this sense includes technology, it is much more than that. Infrastructure includes:

- the design and development of clear, integrated leadership roles and responsibilities;
- appropriate spans of control and staffing;
- the creation of efficient and standardized business processes that support care delivery;
- disciplined, integrated clinical processes that ensure cost-effective delivery of quality care; and
- mechanisms to ensure the engagement of all staff and the development of core competencies to achieve excellence.

By building the infrastructure in this manner healthcare organizations will align the whole enterprise to support ongoing retention and recruitment. Whether management training is increased, positions are shifted, or new recruitment sources are tapped, the infrastructure is critical to success (see Figure 5.1).

For any organization we know that effective recruitment is essential to continued success, but even more critical is retention. In Chapter 1 we described some of the factors leading to undesirable turnover—the flip side of retention. We noted intense frustration with heavy workloads, lack of equipment and essential supplies, perceived incompetence of colleagues and lack of teamwork, etc. These frustrations clearly get in the way of staff's ability to do their work even under the best of circumstances. Add large spans of control and inadequate leadership to this and we have the ingredients for continued turnover.

Although we need to intervene across many fronts quickly, it stands to reason that we begin at the most critical place first: the design and development of clear, integrated leadership roles and responsibilities. It is in the design of pivotal leadership roles that the essential building blocks of infrastructure reside. But even before we tackle the issue of role design we need to be mindful of the propensity of all roles, including leadership roles, to devolve. If we don't understand how this law of organizational entropy works, we'll continue to design roles with lofty purpose and find

Figure 5.1: Elements of an Effective Infrastructure

1. Appropriate distribution of strategic, operational, and tactical responsibility across all roles
2. Appropriate staffing and span of control
3. Efficient and standardized business processes that support care delivery
4. Disciplined, integrated clinical processes that ensure cost-effective delivery of quality care
5. Mechanisms to ensure the engagement of all employees and the development of core competencies to achieve excellence.

---

that, time and again, they wind up being executed in ways that don't look anything like we intended.

KEEPING ROLES FROM DEVOLVING

In any job, including leadership roles, there are three broad types of activities (all of which are important) that have different effects on organizational performance. These can be thought of in terms of rungs on a ladder, building on each other. At the base are day-to-day tactical activities, in the middle are operational activities, and at the top are strategic activities. Assuming the activities are appropriate, tactically focused activity addresses short-term issues that need to get done to move the enterprise forward now, such as responding to the needs of staff, physicians, and patients; securing equipment; meeting an emergent regulatory issue; completing budgets; and responding to requests for information. Tactical activity often entails the adrenaline rush associated with solving today's crisis. To the extent it leaves staff feeling good about "doing something" it tends to be self-reinforcing. But, as we'll see later in this chapter, this type of activity doesn't move the enterprise forward.

This is not to suggest that tactical activity isn't important. It is, and all jobs have elements that are tactical.

At the operational level are intermediate-type activities that are focused on improving the processes that govern and control tactical-level activity. Such activities include, for example, quality improvement initiatives; meetings designed to improve cross-functional collaboration; and training aimed at enhancing decision-making processes and individual skills in critical thinking, negotiation, and conflict management. These mid-range activities are critical to the current and future success of the organization. Failure to engage effectively in cross-functional collaboration means that delivery of care isn't seamless. Failure of support areas in delivering what their internal customers require undermines patient care, patient satisfaction, and employee morale. Ineffective unit-based processes create unnecessary activity—too many hand-offs, not enough coordination, rework, etc.—that puts more time into the realm of the tactical and increases costs to deliver service.

At the strategic level are activities focused on the future. Because they are future focused they are essential to the continued success of the enterprise. Strategic activities include such things as succession planning, building the leadership competencies for tomorrow's (in three to five years) leaders, defining critical roles for tomorrow, proactively managing the culture, building an environment for excellence and ensuring accountability for excellence, identifying new service/business opportunities, redesigning core business processes, planning the workforce, and investing in technology to support radical (and nonradical) change in process to optimize clinical outcomes, efficiency, effectiveness, etc.

Clearly, some positions operate at one level a greater percentage of the time than do others. Technical and support staff, by design, spend most of their time executing at the tactical level. Executives should be spending the greatest portion of their time at the strategic level. The ultimate key to success is to ensure appropriate balance across all three categories of activity.

The Challenge of Balancing Levels of Responsibility

Unfortunately, there is a tendency for all positions across all industries to migrate down to tactical activity. The crush of daily demands and attempts to be responsive (that is, reactive) to immediate customer requests puts pressure on even the best-intended to stay balanced. One senior healthcare executive described the following story to us in a rather embarrassed tone to illustrate the point.

In an attempt to control costs he and his colleagues were asked to enforce a new policy from the finance department. Hospital operations blessed the policy, which required the following controls: All expenses, including those budgeted, were to be countersigned by the executive over the area. Thus, the executive found himself approving $100 toner purchases for existing printers! Not exactly a good use of his time. For him to approve the expense as "legitimate" he needed to review the request with the manager in question. Doing the review took a day or two, given everyone's busy schedules. The fact that the manager's judgment was not trusted was a morale issue, and the process of control slowed down legitimate work. Given that this was just one of too many such policies to tighten controls, the executive didn't have a whole lot of time left to plan for tomorrow. If he wasn't doing it, then who was? In this same institution, managers were busy plugging holes as staffing gaps threatened quality (and the basic safety) of care.

Making phone calls to cajole nurses (and others) to come in to work has become commonplace in the industry over the last several years. This is not saying that adequate staffing isn't important. It is critical! But when managers are engaged regularly in such triage activity, something is seriously amiss. What has happened is that broken processes (operational-level activity), in part brought about by insufficient planning and anticipating (strategic-level activity), have created a series of crises at the tactical level, diverting attention away from real prevention. One of the most vivid and disturbing illustrations of this is the revolving recruitment/retention door we see at all too many healthcare institutions. As one prominent healthcare executive at a major university medical center remarked: "We're doing an excellent job recruiting qualified staff. The only problem is that we lose them faster than we bring them in. And it's been going on this way for over a year." So everyone is involved in the "staffing drill."

At some level, tactically focused activity is very rewarding for most people. Most people like checking things off of the list so that at the end of the day, they can feel they've accomplished something. Then there's the adrenaline rush of putting out the local fires; fire prevention (operational-level activity) usually doesn't have the same satisfaction (or recognition) associated with it. Future-focused activity isn't concrete. It's complex, it takes time, it doesn't show immediate results. It's grey. But by failing to carve out significant time for thinking clearly about issues, their root causes, and their solutions, planning and building infrastructure for tomorrow's challenges will not occur. We will only be left with revolving doors and broken processes.

Systemic Causes of Role Devolution

The propensity of roles to devolve to the tactical is in proportion to an organization's tendency to be reactive and to maintain a short-term financial emphasis without paying balanced attention to other critical strategic drivers such as quality, employee satisfaction, and customer satisfaction. This is not to suggest that being financially responsive is inappropriate. Rather, it is the failure to integrate multiple forces, the inability to balance competing demands without sacrificing the needs of any one group, and the lack of focus on tomorrow while managing today that accelerate the tendency of roles to devolve and ultimately move to crisis situations. Take, for instance, the following situations that highlight the complexity of the problem and its seemingly intractable nature.

A healthcare executive of one of the top-100 hospitals in our survey commented that for years she had been dissatisfied with the manner in which nurse managers executed their jobs, despite their reasonably well-articulated job description. There was wide variance in skill and ability among them, and admittedly they had little formal development/coaching and very broad spans of control. She believed that part of the problem was the corporate office's confusion over which customers the group should respond to—patients, families, physicians, or employees. Further, she reasoned that until the corporate office decided on the priority for focus it appeared likely that her staff would be left no choice but to lurch from one customer set to another. The ability to balance and reconcile competing priorities was clearly not a strong suit for this executive, and the accountabilities had not been clearly defined.

Complicating the nurse managers' situation was the fact that support areas, such as materials, pharmacy, and transport, had cut back their level of support to internal customers (that is, the nursing management) in an attempt to reduce cost. The following incident in this institution vividly describes a situation we hear repeatedly across the country that highlights the failure of support areas to provide support. A senior RN was missing equipment needed to deliver patient care on her unit. She reported the problem repeatedly to her manager, but her manager was unable to get supplies delivered in a reliable and predictable manner. So once again the RN called down to the materials department to obtain the missing equipment. She was then rudely informed that she would need to send someone down from the floor to pick it up because materials was once again short staffed. And so she did, rather than demand that materials fulfill its support mission to the floor. This example of tolerance for broken systems, making do, and covering for other areas is altogether too common. To illustrate just how bad it can get, we heard continuous reports of "search and recover" and "search and hoard" missions that are aimed at retrieving or "stealing" enough supplies and equipment to make it through the shift.

Not that there had not been attempts to address these problems. Indeed in this same hospital a committee studied the problem of "disappearing equipment" for over a year and came up with a set of recommendations, including attaching some of the more elusive devices to the wall! When asked what happened to the suggestions, we learned nothing. The chair of the group left, and with him apparently went the solutions. No one took up the cause afterward, no one demanded accountability for the time the committee spent, and no one formalized the recommendations into a report. But the problems and the associated frustrations remained.

A variety of factors conspire to force patient care managers to allocate their time to the tactical. These factors stem from a short-term financial focus and a reactive approach to planning and customer satisfaction. In concrete terms, we see a shortage of line personnel, most notably clinical staff; unwieldy spans of control with limited supervisory or leadership substructure to delegate to; support departments that are also short staffed and not held accountable for making patient care support their first priority; and organizational pressures to participate in a variety of broad-based task groups and committees that pull managers away from their primary business. Most people in management positions have been promoted up from the ranks. Their comfort zone lies in the tactical. They have had little or no management development, and most have little opportunity to be exposed to strong management from whom they can learn by example. They also are under pressure from many of their employees to roll up their sleeves and do "real" work.

The net result of the factors described above (i.e., limited resources, little development, staff pressure, and personal satisfaction) encourages managers at all levels to think and behave more tactically than they should for the future viability of their organizations. As one manager aptly stated, "we have met the enemy, and the enemy is us."

DEFINING STRATEGIC, OPERATIONAL, AND
TACTICAL RESPONSIBILITIES

Getting out of the quagmire—moving from a tactical or operational focus to a strategic focus—is no easy task and requires large-scale role redefinition. The biggest challenge is knowing where and how to intervene in what is clearly a multifaceted, systemic problem that has significant cultural implications. Knowing where to start the journey to bring about lasting change is critical. Beginning at the core of the problem and working out from there is the best way to leverage scarce resources. If healthcare delivery and direct patient care are the primary business of the organization, then the pivotal role where all resources and processes converge to make this business happen is the natural starting point: the role of the patient care manager, traditionally the nurse manager.

Arguably, the role of patient care manager is key in providing patient care at any hospital. Given the central thesis of this book, it is only fitting that rebuilding an appropriate infrastructure for tomorrow's healthcare organization starts with the pivotal role of this manager. By systematically redefining the strategic priorities of the role of patient care manager and addressing what incumbents need to fulfill the role—competencies, support systems, staff, management interfaces, etc.—an organization can begin to shift the functioning of the entire enterprise. Let us take a look at how this works through a highly structured process that we call job charter and competency development.

Job Charter and Competency Development

The first step in defining strategic priorities is to challenge the respective assumptions currently held by the organization and patient care managers regarding their role. The method for doing so is to create a job charter, define corresponding competencies, and identify the issues that need to be addressed to successfully implement the charter. This is a formidable but doable task.

A job charter for a given class of jobs—in this case the patient care manager (nurse or other first-line clinical staff)—spells out the critical outcomes that incumbents are responsible for delivering and the ways these expectations contribute to the strategic goals of the organization. When complete, a job charter shines the spotlight on the criticality of the role. It specifies the strategic relevance, position duties and responsibilities, key accountabilities, key interfaces, and decision-making authority of the new position (see Figure 5.2). Competencies define in detail the behavioral outcomes that job incumbents must be capable of delivering with predictability—outcomes that are critical for the achievement of overall business success.

Compared with traditional job descriptions, charters offer a more future-oriented, cross-functional view of the job. Rather than a detailed list of today's tactics, a job charter defines the "big" responsibilities that are critical to long-term success. A job charter process takes into consideration how the environment is changing, examining not only present needs but also what the future environment will require. In healthcare, competition and cost pressures are likely to continue along with shorter hospital stays and patients who are more acutely ill than in the past. Average patient age will increase, and patients will continue to be channeled into ambulatory care and outpatient centers. At the same time, consumers will demand more and payers will expect more data-based results. The inputs and outcomes of the process are represented visually in Figure 5.3. Against this backdrop, the job-charter process forces people to define what the position should be like, to articulate what should be different, and to examine what support is needed for a successful transition.

The heart of the process is not the job-charter document itself but the involvement of patient care managers, directors, and other administrators in redefining what the pivotal job of unit management should entail. The charter is not a predetermined program,

Figure 5.2: Defining Job Charters and Competencies

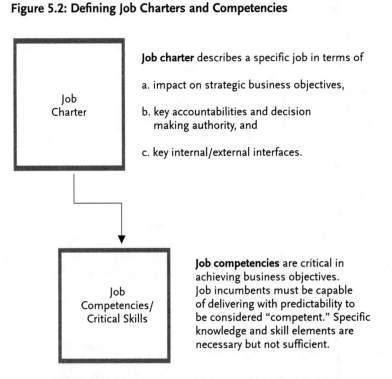

Job charter describes a specific job in terms of

a. impact on strategic business objectives,

b. key accountabilities and decision making authority, and

c. key internal/external interfaces.

Job competencies are critical in achieving business objectives. Job incumbents must be capable of delivering with predictability to be considered "competent." Specific knowledge and skill elements are necessary but not sufficient.

Source: Reprinted with permission from Numerof & Associates, Inc. "Developing Job Charters and Competencies." © 1992–2003. St. Louis, MO: NAI.

suggested and enforced by senior management, but a solution the players are actively engaged in crafting. Not surprisingly, buy-in increases dramatically with such structured engagement. See Figure 5.4 for an example of a job charter.

The following are the kinds of changes that have typically been made to the patient care manager role as a result of the job charter process:

1. more focus on their role as small business managers, including accountability for establishing and articulating program/unit vision, philosophy, and objectives; and
2. multidimensional accountability for clinical, financial, human resources, and patient/customer satisfaction outcomes.

Figure 5.3: Inputs and Outputs of Job Charters and Competencies

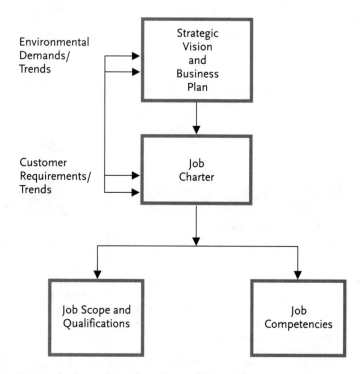

Source: Reprinted with permission from Numerof & Associates, Inc. "Developing Job Charters and Competencies." © 1992–2003. St. Louis, MO: NAI.

Given these changes in the role of the manager, what are the implications for other core operational roles, or more specifically, what should these other roles look like?

BUILDING A LEADERSHIP INFRASTRUCTURE

According to our work with healthcare organizations over the last two decades and in light of current financial pressures and changes in practice, several trends appear to have remained constant. Regardless of who is in management roles, certain leadership responsibilities still need to be done.

Figure 5.4: Example of a Job Charter: Patient Services Manager at Yale-New Haven Hospital

Strategic Relevance

Patient Service Managers [PSM] are responsible for a defined functional area of patient services and must collaborate with others to achieve the hospital's strategic objectives and mission: patient service, teaching, research, and community service. The PSM serves as the direct link between hospital strategies and the staff on the patient care team.

Position Duties and Responsibilities

- Ensuring that desired clinical outcomes are achieved through cost-effective and efficient processes.
- Achieving seamless delivery of service by appropriately involving colleagues, physicians, other customers, and staff to ensure commitment, communication, and cross-functional linkage.
- Collaborating in developing and implementing processes that achieve strategically relevant quality outcomes in a specific functional area.

Key Accountabilities

- Collaborates with division and unit leadership to design, develop, and implement clinically and fiscally responsive program philosophies, goals, and objectives.
- Provides vision and leadership to staff in a collaborative environment that offers job satisfaction and recognition, and stimulates innovative thinking to accomplish goals and objectives.
- Develops customer services standards reflecting excellence consistent with hospital policy for internal/external customers in collaboration with unit leadership and appropriate departments.
- In conjunction with division leadership, establishes and manages a process for monitoring and controlling staff turnover by unit, title, and type.

Key Interfaces

External: The PSM interacts *primarily* with such external interfaces as physicians and patients and secondarily with professional counterparts and vendors/suppliers.

Internal: The PSM interacts *primarily* with such internal interfaces as other PSMs and divisional leadership and *secondarily* with such internal interfaces as non-division directors and other hospital staff.

Decision-Making Authority

To formulate and execute unit/program vision, goals and plans consistent with hospital strategies and policy [and to] determine whether needed resources have been committed and facilitate the acquisition of additional resources where indicated.

Source: Reprinted with permission from "Nursing in Turmoil: Nurse Managers Redefine Their Roles and Responsibilities," by R. Numerof, M. Abrams, and P. S. Fitzsimons, in *COR Clinical Excellence,* published by COR Healthcare Resources. Copyright 2000. All rights reserved. Reproduction of this excerpt is prohibited without consent from COR Healthcare Resources, Santa Barbara, California (www.corhealth.com).

- New staff members need to be selected and hired, oriented, developed to ensure optimal clinical competency, regardless of their field of practice. This educational challenge is formidable.
- To ensure that clinical practice is current and responsive in adapting to shifts in standards and changes in technology, focus on advanced clinical practice is needed.
- Beyond advanced practice and educational support, process improvement must be performed as well.

The critical question is how to structure this work to provide optimal effectiveness, keeping in mind serious financial constraints. Should the work be structured so that separate individuals with distinct titles perform them? Or should this work be integrated into one role? Although arguments can be made on both sides, our experience suggests that in today's complex environment, splitting out these roles so that there is distinct ownership and accountability for each is preferable in most circumstances. This is true despite the increased overhead coordination costs associated with having separate individuals play these roles. Creating clear boundaries for a given role (e.g., leading process improvement, providing educational support, or ensuring focus on advanced clinical practice) must be done in such a way that the roles must have enough breadth. In this way, these newly defined positions will remain interesting and challenging yet maintain organizational flexibility and provide enough structure to promote operational efficiency.

Let's explore the rationale for creating distinct roles. First, clear boundary definition increases the likelihood of focus. Focus, in turn, makes it easier to tie accountability to results, minimizing the tendency in all organizations of overhearing such things as "I didn't get to x since I was pulled in to do y." Given the problem of role entropy, distinctness makes it easier to ensure the strategic and operational focus of the role, thus serving as an antidote to the tactical pulls that undermine overall effectiveness. Where the work is more stable and the required disciplines more firmly established, it might be conceivable to integrate these disparate functions into one role. Unfortunately, this is not the case in healthcare today.

What follows is a discussion of four roles that need to be clarified: education, advanced practice support, process improvement, and administrative support. Each of these roles supports the manager in very specific ways. In addition, we explore one additional role that offers local managerial support: the role of shift or clinical manager.

Education Role

For nursing services, the role of education has long been recognized as critical in the ongoing development of clinical practice competence. Whether from the perspective of mandatory education or the introduction of new technology, nursing staffs have generally seen the value of such learning. Until relatively recently, the primary focus of such learning had been almost exclusively nurses, and those who provided the learning had been designated clinical nurse educators (CNEs), a position that has had some considerable longevity in the field. Deployment of CNEs typically took one of two forms—centralized to ensure consistency and efficiency in providing general orientation and mandatory education or decentralized to enable local education efforts to be better matched to perceived local needs. The latter form of educators were frequently known as UBEs or unit-based educators. Once again, their purview was nursing staff—new grads, new equipment/procedure introduction, etc.

The narrow, nursing-only focus is problematic in today's environment given that non-RN staff who are engaged in patient care support need development and typically fall through the cracks. The complexity of the care delivery environment makes an entirely centralized or decentralized structure not workable. To add to the challenges in the current environment, new grads and to some extent new employees are assigned to preceptors—teaching roles that were heavily introduced throughout the 1980s to help facilitate the transition of the novice nurse. Philosophically, all nurses with experience typically were expected to serve as preceptors and bring along their less-experienced colleagues. The assumption underlying this principle was that serving as a preceptor was an exercise in leadership that all should discharge. The problems associated with the typical preceptor-based training in healthcare are those that you would see anytime new employees are expected to learn a complex task through decentralized, unstructured on-the-job training as described below.

The All-Serve-As-A-Preceptor Model

Unfortunately, the intensity of healthcare delivery today has exacerbated the flaws inherent in the all-serve-as-a-preceptor model. First, precious little, if any, consistent development has been given to staff on what it takes to be a good preceptor. Thus, individual preceptors are free to figure it out on their own, offering little consistency in approach or quality. Second, preceptors and their preceptees may not have a consistent relationship over time—that is, they will inevitably work different shifts. Third, few institutions require formalized, regular, constructive feedback on preceptors' performance. Fourth, preceptors rarely get feedback on their effectiveness. Perhaps most problematic with this educational model is the fact that preceptors teach "their practice," which leads to non-standard clinical approaches.

New staff members are often severely criticized for their technique by a new preceptor and told that what they learned yesterday is not the correct approach today. Add to this the organization's tendency to throw inexperienced staff into the staffing mix prematurely to cover staffing vacancies and we have the making for high turnover among new staff early in their tenure. Furthermore, the criteria for being judged "ready" are often not explicit, and competencies are almost never evaluated in an objective, systematic manner. Because orientees frequently have multiple preceptors, being judged "ready" most often comes down to whether any of the preceptors (i.e., experienced personnel) have any red flags to report. In the absence of any reported red flags, the orientee is assumed to be ready.

So what are more optimal solutions to this dilemma of responding to a situation in which increasing numbers of inexperienced staff need to be trained and developed rapidly while ensuring competency and safe deployment? Let's tackle the problem of educational structure and deployment first and then revisit the preceptor role in the context of that structure.

Alternative Models

The structure and delivery of any effective training program follows certain principles of educational design. In turn, needs assessment, development of a curriculum architecture, and course/program evaluation all have distinct methodologies and professionally recognized optimal ways of being performed. To expect that such technical proficiency is universally distributed to all educators in a given facility is probably unrealistic. But not to have such discipline in all educational endeavors is a missed opportunity. The challenge then is how to build this capability and deploy it in a cost-effective manner. Two approaches stand out as good examples of a solution to this complex set of problems. Although neither is perfect in its implementation, both offer insight into what can be accomplished even in a large, complex, urban medical center. The more unusual approach is the adjunct faculty model, while the other is the integrated matrix model.

In the adjunct faculty model, relatively few full-time curriculum designers perform needs assessment and "manufacture" the courseware supplemented by contract extenders as needed. The content covers all mandatory education, orientation, and general clinical updates and is delivered by "adjunct faculty." This adjunct faculty is composed of hospital employees—that is, practicing clinicians from various units/programs who are subject matter experts and have interest/capability in teaching. They have been given training in facilitation and presentation/delivery. In one large university medical center, approximately eight designers are mapped to specific areas of content work with approximately 38 adjunct faculty.

This model is not dissimilar to the scientific training approach employed by AstraZeneca, a pharmaceutical company, where a small number of training staff design highly technical, product-specific training mapped by therapeutic area. The structure of this model is compelling for two reasons. First, highly technical expertise (i.e., needs assessment, design, evaluation) is centralized in a core group of experts, which ensures efficiency, effectiveness, and consistency of approach. Second, clinical delivery is offered by locally recognized and credible subject matter experts, creating an optimal learning environment. The challenge here is in having sufficient delivery experts and/or taking them out of staffing to meet the growing demand for clinical education.

By way of contrast, the integrated matrix model (also employed by a large urban university medical facility) works with a much larger contingent of educators, some of whom focus on large-scale organizational programming and mandatory education and the remainder address the needs of local units/clinical programs. Centrally managed to ensure consistency of methodology and approach, these unit-based educational staff members are deployed to support the needs of their internal clients. Part of the leadership complement of the units they support, they enjoy a matrix management model: they report to their central manager for technically related matters and to their program manager for responsiveness and effectiveness of learning interventions. In all cases, they carry a minimal clinical load to remain current and clinically credible, not to fill vacancies. Because they are part of the units they support, frequently these local educators are perceived to be more responsive.

Both of the models offered here for consideration rely on a strong centralized core of technical expertise. Important organizational design considerations drive this perspective. Whenever there is highly specialized technical expertise that an organization needs to deploy, that expertise tends to be kept together to ensure technical freshness because the experts challenge each other. Diffusing such expertise tends to dilute it over time, unless the expertise is (or will become) a core competence of the entire organization. In the case of education design, this is clearly not the intent.

Having discussed structure and deployment, let us revisit the structural implications for preceptors and the key accountabilities for the clinical educator.

Defining Accountabilities for Preceptors and Clinical Educators

As educational activity requires technical design and specialized expertise, so too does effective coaching and orientation of new staff. Assuming that managers' span of control and focus in today's environment preclude them from directly engaging in this level of support, then someone else needs to assume the responsibility (but in a manner very different from how it is done in most organizations today). A limited number of preceptors tied to specific clinical practice areas and that report to the manager in charge will be certified as preceptors. Selected because of their clinical expertise and innate desire to impart knowledge to others, they will be taken through a time-limited program designed to give them the requisite skills to do their precepting. Such a program will focus on the essentials of providing timely, specific, and usable positive and negative feedback; engaging in structured lessons-learned discussions; etc. The ultimate objective is to create a learning environment that strives for and achieves excellence in practice. Competency-based evaluation of the preceptee provides consistency among preceptors, while preceptee ratings of preceptors provide data to enhance the performance of preceptors. The preceptor program can be set up and facilitated through the central education function to ensure organizational alignment and consistency across the board.

Preceptors will be part of the local clinical team, reporting to the unit or program manager and serving as part of its leadership complement. Preceptors will carry a clinical load, but this load (the actual number of patients) will vary depending on the number of preceptees, their expertise, and the complexity of care being delivered on the unit/program. With this type of design local needs will be met in the service of overall organizational excellence.

Before we leave this section we need to explore briefly the key accountabilities and primary focus of our clinical educators. Our central educators clearly need curriculum architecture and course design competency as well as needs assessment and evaluation expertise. To the extent that these designers are also pulled into delivery, they must have good platform training capabilities as well. Consistent with the models we are recommending, our unit-based educators or adjunct faculty must have solid clinical skills, excellent platform skills, and the ability to translate new clinical approaches and procedural change in such a way that ensures buy-in and new behavior. The ability to manage change and work through resistance to adopting new approaches is key to success. At the local level, these individuals will be expected to assess local needs in concert with the manager to whom they report and other members of the unit/program leadership. Working with clinical experts, they will engage in translating advances in practice to day-to-day activity to maintain practice excellence. They will also be engaged in reviewing current practice to identify gaps and in designing and delivering solutions for local remediation (e.g., blood pressure reading accuracy, medication administration accuracy, infection management, etc.). Thus, the local clinical educator must be a diagnostician of learning needs for the clinical area they support, a designer of local solutions (with the assistance of central educational resources), and a recognized clinician.

One last point must be emphasized. We have been silent on the audience for these educators and preceptors. Our very strong opinion is that these individuals need to own the ongoing educational needs of the clinical teams they support. If, for example, patient care technicians, patient care assistants, nurses aides, etc. are part of the mix, then educators need to assume responsibility for the learning and competency of these groups (in addition to their responsibility for the ongoing learning of the nursing staff, which has heretofore been their sole purview). Only with this approach can excellence across the board be achieved.

Advanced Practice Support Role

In an age of continuously advancing technology and more complexly ill patients, no healthcare organization can remain still. For the top hospitals, one of the continuing challenges is how to anticipate changes in clinical practice based on new technology and/or research findings. This is no easy task. Although this is less of an issue for rehab and acute nontertiary care facilities, it should be of prime concern for those organizations that emphasize the care of highly diverse and complex cases—in particular, teaching institutions and university-affiliated medical centers. The critical question for any healthcare organization is how to ensure that tomorrow's practice becomes mainstream as rapidly as possible. Together with clinical consultation around highly complex patients, this is the domain of the advanced clinical practitioner.

Although the need for an advanced practice clinician seems instinctively obvious at some level, it is a role associated with a fair degree of controversy in the nursing profession in particular. The historical roots of the role within nursing lie in the clinical nurse specialist (CNS) role, an advanced-practice position. Typically this role requires master's-level preparation at a minimum and is focused on a particular patient population or disease (e.g., geriatric, pediatric, oncology, cardiopulmonary, etc.). Over the years, incumbents have been engaged in developing clinical care pathways with physicians and other relevant care specialists. In the model we are proposing, we envision the role of the advanced practice clinician (APC) as a consultant primarily to the unit/program manager(s) he or she is mapped to support. APCs will also serve as members of the leadership team of that unit and are also engaged as clinical consultants by the staff of that program around the needs of complex patient care.

Many hospitals have attempted to implement advanced practice roles, but the results have been often disappointing. These roles have generated a lot of friction between program managers and the advanced practitioner and between educators and the advanced practitioner. At the root of the friction has been the confusion between managerial authority and clinical expertise. Specifically, some managers have been willing to delegate/abdicate responsibility for the clinical competence of their staff to the APC (or CNS). Staff members have looked to the CNS for guidance without an understanding of who's really "running the program." In some cases, the APC role devolves into an educational role to fill a gap in practice, leaving a hole in defining and delivery of future competencies. Clearly, the role of the APC is needed, in which the APC works with his or her educational partner to identify emerging and current needs and consults in the process, content, and delivery of this material. To be effective, this role requires high levels of collaboration and the ability to work through gray areas and to recognize that, at the end of the day, accountability for staff performance is still the domain of the program/unit manager.

Process-Improvement Role

For many years, healthcare organizations (whether inpatient or outpatient, acute, rehab, or critical care) have engaged in some form of process-improvement activity. In years past, this activity has fallen under the heading of continuous quality improvement; total quality management; process redesign or reengineering; process improvement; and process excellence or, in some institutions, "Six Sigma." The purpose behind each of these approaches is essentially the same: identify critical outcomes for key customer groups, take non-value-added activity (and personnel) out of the process, and reduce cost of delivering the outputs of the process while improving output quality. It is beyond the scope of this book to talk about the relative merits of these approaches. Suffice it to say, however, that systematically improving core processes across the organization must be a continuous focus for all institutions, regardless of their size, location, and type of care delivery. To the extent that standardized core business and clinical processes (e.g., admission and discharge, basic assessment, customer satisfaction, equipment/supplies cleanliness, etc.) can be defined across the whole enterprise with unit-specific processes built on top of the general base, dramatic improvements in quality and efficiency can be made.

Most healthcare organizations have centralized some process-improvement activity but few have built and imbedded the necessary discipline to make process improvement the way business is done. Although clinical pathways, for example, have been introduced widely, the extent to which they are systematically followed is quite another matter. Clearly, focus on and commitment to process improvement must be a central consideration in the development of leadership infrastructure. How best to structure this critical work is the issue at hand.

Central responsibility for organizationwide process improvement was evident in most of the top-100 hospitals in our survey. How well the technology associated with the function was deployed depended on the particular institution. As an organizing principle, the central approach does have real utility, if we keep in mind the key responsibilities of the function. For example, defining a common methodology for structuring and managing process-improvement projects, analyzing data, deriving the cost-benefit of potential changes, and implementing change are extremely beneficial from an efficiency and effectiveness perspective. By taking responsibility for educating relevant participants, we minimize the costs associated with one-time projects and the expense of reinventing methodology. Given that many such projects are either organizationwide or have organizationwide implications, central and common methodology enables continuity across projects and can minimize duplication of effort such as in every unit inventing its own unique approach to "x." One of the important but frequently overlooked opportunities for the central functions to fulfill is the capture and systematic deployment of best practices, an opportunity we see throughout the industry.

But what about the unit-specific or program-specific needs for improvement, especially given that the manager in our model for the future is accountable for building in continuous improvement as a core unit/program activity? Clearly, a need exists at the unit level for focused accountability for (1) implementing organizationwide initiatives and (2) initiating, implementing, and monitoring unit-specific initiatives. Leading these projects is a critically important job that requires knowledge of relevant process-improvement methodology, effective skills in project management, and an understanding of change management. Who is in a position to provide this guidance at the unit level and how should these important leadership roles be deployed? To ensure credibility among unit peers and the program, the incumbent assigned the responsibility for leading such initiatives should have clinical and technical expertise that reflects the core competency of the unit. The number of staff expected to lead such initiatives depends on the size of the program/unit in question and the number of initiatives required. The rule of thumb, however, is less is more, which is clearly an orientation that is contrary to existing practice in most institutions where it is not uncommon to require all staff members to lead such projects. Although structured broad participation in such initiatives is highly desirable, expecting everyone to lead one suggests that all candidates for these roles have the ability and the desire to do so. This is a naïve assumption at best and also suggests that no special skills are required for success. For most programs, having one or two really skilled individuals is optimal, with the idea of developing backfill talent through active participation in such projects.

Administrative Support Role

When asked the question "what will make your jobs easier?" surveyed managers across the country consistently rated the need for administrative support as a high priority. In the last ten years, one of the easiest cost-elimination tactics was the abolishment of administrative support, which was rationalized in part by the introduction of computers. Essentially, the concept behind it was if you can type directly into the computer, why would you need an administrative assistant anyway? Although the decision may have made sense then, today's environment places even more administrative burden on managers, taking away precious time they can ill afford to give up to deliver tasks and activity that can be provided at a much-lower cost structure. Scheduling and coordinating myriad meetings, managing minutes, filing, ordering equipment, and gathering and entering data are just a few administrative activities that consume managers' precious time.

To address this problem, some facilities have attempted to provide centralized administrative support in the form of secretarial pools that consist of nondedicated staff. Although the concept sounds good on paper, and the cost is certainly appealing to many, in reality these secretarial pools have not been effective solutions to the need for administrative support. Lack of dedicated staff undermines work ownership and tends to degrade the quality of document production. It also undermines support staff's identification with the work and hence the facility. Those situations in which pools work are designed in such a way that there is primary mapping of staff to a particular manager or set of managers with the understanding that work overflow will be picked up by members of the support team as needed. But work identity isn't the only problem with pools. In addition, the physical logistics of getting memos, reports, and graphics back and forth have proven to be an obstacle to using these services. Filing, scheduling, and summarizing meeting minutes as well as some data entry and graphic presentations don't get done at all because of the lack of physical proximity. This simply makes the service too much trouble. As an indication of just how much administrative burden is absorbed by managers, activity studies done by NAI revealed that between 12 and 18 percent of managers' time was spent in performing clearly administrative functions. And these findings came from stronger managers in high-profile, highly rated top-100 institutions.

Competency is another issue in considering the problem of administrative support in building the leadership infrastructure. Some institutions believe that the traditional unit clerk is optimally positioned to provide any of the support functions required. However, on deeper reflection, this role may not be a good fit for the problem at hand. Visibly, the unit clerk (or whatever the title may be) is at the center of unit activity, answering questions about a patient's status from anxious family members who have just arrived; receiving flowers for patients; putting together charts and pulling them; answering the phone; contacting staff and other units; attempting to track down equipment and supplies; sometimes running down to lab and x-ray; and trying to appear cool, calm, and collected amidst the hectic activity of a typical day. Even if the unit clerk has the time to provide needed administrative support to the manager (which is unlikely given the job description above), the question regarding skill level remains. The unit clerk is an entry-level position and as such is associated with lower pay. It is also first and foremost a reception job, and thus incumbents do not typically have the analytic and technical skills required for the administrative support functions needed. This is not to suggest that the role of unit clerk is not important. Quite the contrary. This suggests that the requirements of administrative support are not being filled; thus they are picked up by the manager, who is then taken away from more strategic and operational functions of their role.

Local Managerial Support Role

Earlier in this chapter we argued that building an infrastructure to support excellence in patient care delivery must begin with the pivotal role of the patient care manager. Following this discussion we argued for clarity in four key and distinct roles to support the manager: education, advanced practice, process improvement, and administrative. None of these roles functions in a managerial capacity, although the former three are clearly part of a "leadership complement" of any unit/program. We have not discussed our recommendations for the role of the local clinical manager, which is the fifth and final role needed to support the manager. Let's explore the need for additional clinical management, beginning with the charge designation.

The charge person has typically been a nurse who assumes the go-to role for a shift. This person sometimes directs traffic flow; frequently responds to staff issues in the absence of the line manager; and serves as the point person for physicians, family members, and patients when they have difficulty locating their nurse or primary caregiver. The assumption surrounding the responsibility of preceptorship (i.e., it's everyone's job to pitch in and do it) all too commonly has been applied to the charge activity. Whether the assumption evolved out of a sense that being a charge is a demanding job (which it is) so no one should be unduly burdened by it or out of a sense that everyone should be given an opportunity to serve is immaterial. The problem of continuously rotating charge should not be underestimated. Just as not everyone makes a good mentor/preceptor, the skills required for excellent performance in the charge role are not universally distributed. These differences aren't lost on staff, physicians, or patients. Staff and others report that when certain people are "on," things run very smoothly; when they are "off," things tend to not run as smoothly. Our interviews with staff nurses from the top-100 hospitals revealed that the picture tended to be the same. Staff put in their charge time because they were required to do so, and some really liked their role and aspired to be managers while others just got by. Given the often dramatic churn of patients in and out of units and the movement of staff, having stability in the charge role is critical for increasing continuity focus, and accountability for excellence. Imagine the natural reluctance of today's in-charge staff person to tackle controversial staff, personnel, equipment, or process issues. This person may think: If I can just make it through the shift, this will be someone else's problem tomorrow! Although the concept of "permanent" charge may not be feasible for all institutions, limiting the role to a very small number of staff members who have competencies to do the job and who receive training will greatly improve process effectiveness in healthcare.

But moving from rotating charge to making it a more permanent position does not solve all of the problems with local managerial support. The charge individual has never been a manager. As such he or she is not able to administer discipline and his or her authority is frequently challenged directly. Not surprisingly, managers (who may not be available at the time) may spend days interviewing staff, tracking down incident reports, and performing other investigative work to get to the facts of the situation that needs disciplinary attention. By the time the employees in question receive their feedback/disciplinary action, weeks have transpired, which is not a particularly effective way of handling problems. But it is not only in dealing with unit staff that lack of authority is an issue. Other healthcare departments are notorious for not delivering on promises, which is a result in part of their own real and perceived staffing shortages. However, the likelihood of getting a positive response increases exponentially when one possesses a management title!

All of this suggests that some form of shift management is needed to focus on tactical issues related to the day-to-day delivery of care on the unit/program. Whether the title is shift or clinical manager, this critical individual, under the direction of the patient care manager, is responsible for ensuring consistent, efficient patient care for a defined shift or smaller unit in a functional area of the hospital.

THE ROLE OF SCARCE RESOURCES

One of the challenges in healthcare today is the ever-present reality of scarce resources. Unfortunately, many hospitals have attempted to deal with these cost pressures by cutting staff and internal services under the guise of redesign. Such decisions frequently reflect silo-based thinking. For instance, in one institution, pharmacy pulled back drug deliveries based on the assumption that nursing services would pick up any needed drugs in off hours. In a similar vein, materials and central stores either stopped deliveries or, in some cases, actually closed shop after 5:00 p.m. The assumption was that supplies would be available and delivered during the day shift, obviating the need for any coverage for evenings and nights. From our experience, we can cite abundant examples that illustrate the lack of responsiveness of environmental services, such as not keeping service-level agreements, allowing quality to be transient, or patients complaining about lack of cleanliness. Human resources departments take their fair share of heat from disgruntled internal customers as well. Most notable here are issues relating to finding qualified candidates and filling positions in a timely manner as well as supporting managers in performance management and discipline issues. Finance is not immune to criticism by patient care areas. Criticisms typically leveled here are related to inadequately detailed reports that create countless hours of manual retroactive review to get answers to variance questions. And the list just goes on. Perhaps most disturbing is the actual failure of clinical departments to respond to codes, which is ostensibly the result, once again, of short staffing.

Of course, support departments may be quick to point the guns in the opposite direction, typically accusing primary clinical departments of arrogance and noncollaboration. Under conditions of scarce resources there is a natural tendency to point a finger and blame someone else—another department, another individual, an administrative policy, etc. At the end of the day, however, blame does not get the finance questions answered, minimize human resources bureaucracy and make them more responsive, make environmental services workers committed to cleanliness, or deliver drugs and supplies when needed. Patient needs must come first, so typically clinical delivery areas are responsible for finding a way to cope with such scarcity!

Although there are clearly exceptions to this, the coping strategy that we have seen typically entailed a "just do it" attitude and the clinical areas covering for the support departments. Laudable? We think not. Given that the scarcity crisis has become normatively acceptable in too many hospitals, we find direct caregivers pulled from caring to running transport; garnering drugs, supplies, and equipment; and in many cases regularly cleaning rooms to cover for inadequate housekeeping services. The environment that is created and too often tolerated is corrosive and clearly dysfunctional. On a short-term basis it is entirely reasonable to expect people to "pitch in and do whatever it takes." The problems we are outlining, however, are not short term. They are systemic and reflect a lack of integrated planning, lack of needed change in core process, and lack of accountability for results. Most importantly they create an unsafe environment for patients and staff. In fact, this environment is the breeding ground for turnover. Based on employee survey data and interviews with thousands of managers in healthcare institutions across the country, these conditions have been cited time and again over the last several years as sources of dissatisfaction and job burnout. With no one listening or no one able to turn things around, people with job options are opting out of the system. What exactly is senior management's role in turning this around?

THE ROLE OF SENIOR MANAGEMENT

Building an effective infrastructure is all about processes, role definition, and accountability. Once in place, who the manager is doesn't really matter. The infrastructure enables staff to focus on the right things to ensure desired outcomes. It's this infrastructure and its associated culture of excellence and accountability that gives GE the ability to continue without its former CEO Jack Welch.

Clearly, if the infrastructure is to be built, it must be the responsibility of senior management. Senior management must be focused on strategy and the operational execution of strategy. As we described earlier in this chapter, there are pressures even on senior management that cause their activities to devolve to the tactical realm. Whether responding to individual physician requests for equipment or signing off on $100 purchases for toner, many senior managers in healthcare find themselves drowning in the same activity that their more junior staff are attempting to navigate. For the current situation to change, senior management must engage differently: create a balance between resolving short-term financial pressures, staffing, and quality issues and anticipating and planning for longer-term stability.

In the name of protecting the jobs of patient caregivers, many institutions drastically cut support services to the bone. What we have found is that the caregivers have often picked up what the support areas were doing, which takes them away from patient care. The resulting frustrations feed their exit from the healthcare system.

One of the assumptions behind this cutting is the belief that if you cut staff, those remaining will eliminate the non-value-added components of a process, enabling them to cover the workload. This belief presumes that (1) there is non-value activity, (2) people know the difference between value-added and non-value activity, and (3) staff will spontaneously choose to deliver the high-value activity. Given that these assumptions haven't materialized, we must focus on senior management to take a more direct interventional approach to addressing these system problems.

A common issue that we have found is that senior managers, in the name of autonomy, are overly willing to take a laissez-faire attitude when it comes to resolving difficulties that their line managers have encountered while getting support from departments such as information services, human resources, materials, and environmental services. It is unfair to expect (and allow) managers to fix broken systems at the unit level when a concerted, organizational response is needed. Recurring system issues need to be resolved in a focused manner at more senior levels in the organization. Mechanisms need to be established to bring up these issues, track them, resolve them, and keep them resolved. Senior managers need to own and resolve these without pointing fingers and affixing blame either at their support colleagues or their mid-level managers.

In a similar vein, it is unreasonable to expect (and allow) each manager to invent one-off solutions to system issues because their unit is altogether "unique." Multiple pilot projects need to be launched with disciplined and focused implementation and evaluation and then rolled out hospital wide. Building in unique cures for an individual unit's ailments can be on top of the more general, universal fix, which eliminates unneeded and expensive duplication. To accomplish this against a cultural mind-set of "we're unique" will require an enormous change in behavior; but as we'll see in Chapter 7, it can be done.

Failing to step-up to the plate under these circumstances reflects an insensitivity to process discipline and the need for standardization. By letting everyone invent their own process, senior management has moved far away from seeing any value in centralization, allowing a "quiet anarchy" to develop in some organizations. By letting every manager Band-Aid their own solution to any process that they find problematic at the unit level and work out conflicts individually, senior management is abdicating its leadership role. Beyond these two areas (that is, facilitating the resolution of cross-functional support issues and standardizing core processes), senior management needs to reexamine its roles relative to physicians. In many organizations we find tactical problem resolution with doctors occurring very frequently at the level of the vice president or administrative director. The question is why. Clearly, physicians are critically important customers and their concerns should be taken seriously. At issue here is why tactically focused issues do not or cannot get resolved at lower levels. The same dynamics that pull other roles into tactical activity are at work here too, encouraging overinvolvement in working things out. One factor that contributes to the situation is the esteemed-physician status associated with such problem resolutions. Another is the fact that many managers and directors do not have the requisite skills to manage these complex interpersonal encounters. Managers are typically not selected with these skills in mind, and there are rarely structured approaches to help them develop these skills. Finally, physicians are likely to want one person to get them what they want. These three dynamics conspire to pull senior managers more closely into more tactical, day-to-day problem resolution with physicians.

For senior management to accomplish the goal of building an infrastructure, clear expectations for change and focus will need to be set, but this is only the beginning. Each will need to look at how various parts of the complex delivery system have been set up to fail, and only then will clarity around solutions make sense. In some cases cutting back on services, shifting clinical programs, and investing in technology to enable new ways of working will be part of the solution. In others, focused ongoing coaching aimed at bringing higher-order analytic problem-solving skills to the table will be needed. This will help managers to connect the dots, focus on priorities, and develop the needed influence and negotiation skills that will increasingly be required to manage complex changes that must be instituted.

CONCLUSION

Attracting and retaining tomorrow's workforce rests on the healthcare organization's ability to build the needed infrastructure. We have argued for the creation of job charters, which is a new way of defining core roles and accountabilities. We have recognized and discussed the fact that all roles tend to devolve from the strategic and operational to the tactical unless we have mechanisms in place to retard such organizational entropy. Beginning with the central role of patient services manager, we identified five critical roles that are necessary for an effective infrastructure: education, advanced clinical support, process improvement, administrative, and local or shift managerial support. Recognizing that much turnover occurs because of the stress associated with poor processes and lack of cross-functional coordination, we explored the problems of scarce resources and the need of support departments to engage fully in systemic solutions. Given the systemic nature of these difficult problems, we argued that it is senior management's responsibility to engage differently: to create a balance between resolving short-term financial pressures, staffing, and quality issues and anticipating and planning for longer-term stability.

REFERENCES

COR Clinical Excellence. 2000. "Nursing in Turmoil: Nurse Managers Redefine Their Roles and Responsibilities," by R. Numerof, M. Abrams, and P. S. Fitzsimons. Santa Barbara, CA: COR Healthcare Resources.

Numerof & Associates, Inc. "Developing Job Charters and Competencies." 1992–2003. St. Louis, MO: NAI.

CHAPTER 6

Cross-Industry Practices: Lessons from the Best

THE ECONOMIC DOWNTURN in the United States is associated with changes in retention and recruitment strategies as well as massive layoffs across the nation. Despite this trend, 80 companies on *Fortune*'s 2002 "100 Best Companies to Work For" list avoided layoffs. It is remarkable that the best of class maintained their commitment to their employees during truly rough economic times by taking a long-term view of their workforce. Instead of layoffs, these companies offered voluntary leaves of absence, cut bonuses, and decreased base pay across the board to avert financial loss. In those cases where layoffs could not be prevented, severance packages that were unusually generous were offered (for example, CISCO Systems offered six months' severance); outplacement services were offered; and compassion through communication was abundant, with frequent updates from CEOs. Astoundingly, the results often included higher production from workers who had received their layoff notices prior to their departure, which was the case with Agilent Technologies, a spin-off of Hewlett Packard (*Fortune* 2002). These companies had fostered loyalty and trust over time, and their employees felt committed through the duration of their remaining employment.

Unfortunately, many healthcare organizations take a short-term view, recruiting and terminating employees based on short-term fluctuations in business. This, in turn, creates a short-term mindset in their employees. It is a view driven by an hourly mentality—that is, working when volumes are up and cutting hours when volumes are down. Without long-term employment commitment, it is not surprising that many healthcare workers feel little loyalty to their employer beyond their current paychecks. Although no employer can guarantee lifelong employment, healthcare can take a lesson from responses of other companies to the serious economic challenges experienced during the recession.

Although healthcare has traditionally lagged behind other industries in addressing the dynamics underlying recruitment and retention issues, there is evidence that this is changing. Fortunately, many of the methods used successfully in other companies to increase retention and maintain leadership positions can be adapted by healthcare organizations. In this chapter, we discuss 11 winning strategies and explore how to apply them to increase a healthcare organization's chances for success in recruiting and retaining desired employees.

WINNING STRATEGIES

Strategy 1: Creating and Leveraging the Brand

Creating brand loyalty among customers and employees alike is a powerful force for the company able to achieve this distinction. Any organization can differentiate itself and become the "brand of choice" for the employees it is trying to attract. Creating and promoting a brand enables that organization to recruit and then retain the employees it needs for future growth. The brand becomes the magnet that pulls in the best employees. The result of this approach is becoming an employer of choice.

This strategy only works when a company has defined its culture and has created a clear value proposition. The value proposition spells out what is unique and special about the organization and why someone would want to do business with it and work for it. The value proposition creates an image. This image must be easily accessed; emotionally appealing; imbedded in all company activity, policy, and communication; and internalized by all employees. It is no small feat, but its outcome will clearly influence recruitment and retention success. For example, Microsoft, Intel, and other leading technology companies have created an image of being challenging and cutting-edge places to work. Their value proposition attracts talented individuals who want to work for a leader and want to be part of this kind of corporate culture. One benefit of this approach is that employees become emotionally vested in the organization, and they become an additional source of recruitment. Even parts of the government understand this powerful dynamic. The U.S. Air Force instituted a program called "We Are All Recruiters." The program encourages current service members to recruit other individuals and to take ownership of a successful organization (*Air Force News* 2000).

Nordstrom's, the retail department store that has long been recognized for its customer-service orientation, goes out of its way to hire service-committed employees. The Walt Disney Company understands that its parks are a total experience that is only made possible by employees who bring enthusiasm and commitment and see themselves as "actors" in that experience. Equipped with intensive training, even street sweepers understand the criticality of their "part." Getting to this point takes vision, commitment, and discipline. In healthcare the leadership of one innovative institution recognized the importance of this journey many years ago. Miami Valley Hospital in Dayton, Ohio, effectively leveraged its tagline—"The region's leader"—to differentiate itself from other hospitals in the area. According to their president, Bill Thornton, the hospital began using this tagline in 1988 for two purposes: (1) to distinguish

Miami Valley Hospital from the competition for the public and (2) to build aspirations in employees' minds to keep them striving toward that goal of making their institution the region's leader. The second reason is just as important as the first because it inspires individuals to do their best and to continue focusing on improvements every day and every year. This tagline, Thornton reported, is also a powerful tool for recruiting because job candidates want to work for the best institution—that is, the region's leader.

Duke University Hospital in Durham, North Carolina, capitalizes on its academic status as the teaching hospital of Duke University Medical School to attract and retain employees. The hospital leverages its academic environment in promoting the organization to those who are motivated by learning and research: Staff members work on "cutting edge" projects, use newly developed procedures, and have the opportunity to participate in developing academic papers. This atmosphere appeals to those who want the excitement of being on the forefront of their field.

Southwest Airlines, the fourth-ranked company in *Fortune's* 100 Best Companies to Work For in 2001 list, has stated that it puts its employees first and customers second because well-treated employees take care of customers. The airline boasts a family atmosphere, a friendly environment where the CEO says "hello" to employees and participates in loading baggage each Thanksgiving day. The result of the company's emphasis on employees is a 7 percent voluntary turnover rate in 1999 (*Fortune* 2001). By the same token, employees at Federal Express Corporation are ingrained in the philosophy of equal treatment for all. FedEx, which is also listed in *Fortune's* 100 Best Companies to Work For in 2001 and 2002, experienced a 7 percent voluntary turnover rate in 1999 and 10 percent in 2000 (*Fortune* 2002). At FedEx, there is no executive dining room, executive offices are modest, no one is given a company car, and the chairman does not have an assigned parking spot. Most part-time workers receive the same benefits as those who work full time.

At Plante & Moran, an accounting firm based in Michigan that was ranked as number 10 on the 2001 *Fortune*'s 100 Best Companies to Work For list and increased to number 7 in 2002, the "partner row" is notably absent. Each staff member has an enclosed office, regardless of status. This firm's turnover rate was about half that experienced at the Big Five national accounting firms in 1999. CISCO Systems, a high-tech company hit hard by the NASDAQ falloff in 2000 to 2002, made both the *Fortune*'s and *Working Mother*'s Best Companies lists in 2001. CISCO continued to be on the 2002 *Fortune* list in the 15th position despite laying off 5,500 people in 2001; it was number 3 in 2001. At CISCO, there are few visible perks for executives. No one flies first class, and there is no executive dining room. To reinforce corporate values and build a common identity, every employee is expected to know and to work to achieve the top initiatives for the year. The same philosophy is used at other organizations, where each employee commits the company's mission statement to memory (*Fortune* 2002). Having the corporation's mission, goals, and objectives emblazoned on people's foreheads, so to speak, creates identity and ownership.

At Baptist Health Care in Pensacola, Florida, a hospital system with approximately 5,300 employees, managers strive to develop a culture that engages and empowers staff. They work with every single employee to make sure the individual understands the role he or she plays in reaching the organizational mission and values of the institution. According to Pam Bilbrey (2002), senior vice president of corporate development at Baptist Health Care, the system actually spends more time on retention than on recruitment, an anomaly in today's healthcare environment. Further, recruitment for every single position in the organization involves peer interviewing, which engages others in the process and creates buy in. Other employees actually become vested in the new recruit and will support that person to ensure success. The psychological result is that others feel accountable for the success of the new employee, and the tangible result is that turnover has been cut in half since peer interviewing was instituted (*Fortune* 2002). Bank of America promotes an environment where employees are valued and recognized for their contributions to the organization and where a team orientation is expected. This philosophy permeates the organization and is reflected in the design of benefit packages, training initiatives, and recognition programs. For its efforts in creating and enforcing this philosophy, Bank of America is rewarded with a high retention rate, even during the employment shortages of the late 1990s.

In a number of companies, commitment to employees is reflected in various aspects of the culture. At Bank of America and Security Benefit Group, individuals are called "associates," not "employees." This, by itself, doesn't ensure desired results but reflects one way that these organizations feel creates an atmosphere of appreciation and support, where employees are valued at the individual level. This relationship between employees and their organizations is what creates a culture that fosters a high focus on customers and quality. According to Tom Breitenbach (2002), chief executive officer of Premier Health Partners, a major healthcare system in Dayton, Ohio, "If employees feel valued and know that their contribution makes a difference, and the organization consistently provides an exceptional working environment, they will reflect their positive perceptions in dealing with patients and their families. PHP continually aims for excellence in health care and then projects that image to the community at large. This makes individuals want to be a part of our team."

Strategy 2: Using Incentives for Specific Groups or Key Talent

Various industries also offer a variety of retention inducements for specific employee groups and key talent. Generally employed on an as-needed basis, these incentives are targeted toward high-demand occupations critical to core operations.

The Philadelphia Board of Education, for example, grants bonuses to teachers who can fulfill a gap in specific courses, including special education, mathematics, chemistry, physics, and Spanish (*Philadelphia Inquirer* 2001). In addition, the board pays annual bonuses, ranging from $1,500 to $2,000, to certified teachers willing to work at particular schools that lack instructors. At AFG Consulting, an information technology consulting group, retention bonuses are project related and are offered at the completion of a project, usually after 18 months (Monster.com 2001). These bonuses vary from $5,000 to $25,000. Although this is a huge incentive for an employee to stay with the company, it isn't always effective in that a larger sign-on bonus from another employer can still lure the employee away prior to project completion.

Bonuses have been offered at hospitals for many years. University of Maryland Medical Center (UMMC) has offered retention bonuses in exchange for a commitment to stay with the organization. According to Ann Regier (2002), director of patient care services at UMMC, these bonuses were implemented as a stop-gap measure prior to restructuring the organization's compensation system. Senior executives recognized the need for some intervention to prevent excessive turnover because of noncompetitive salaries. Although the system was undergoing redesign, UMMC offered staff-retention bonuses as a short-term fix until an improved compensation system could be implemented. These bonuses were structured to be paid four times over an 18-month period. If the employee left the hospital for any reason, the employee was expected to pay back the bonus. The intent was to get employees to make a commitment to the hospital and become a "partner" in implementing upcoming changes. Results were good: about 80 percent of nursing staff participated in the retention bonus program. Although UMMC planned to eliminate these bonuses once compensation changes were made and long-term solutions were implemented, other institutions were ramping up such bonuses. In some parts of the country, for example, retention bonuses for critical care nurses exceeded $10,000 per year for three years. Such approaches provide short-term relief to an ongoing issue, and thus, are not "solutions" to the problem of retention, something recognized by the very institutions that use them.

Miami Valley Hospital (MVH) also provides retention bonuses in the form of "tuition buy back." According to Barbara Smith (2002), director of human resources, this program is offered to nurses who have graduated recently and have reached one year of employment with MVH. For three years, nurses are granted up to $3,000 per year to assist in paying back qualified student loans, which is quite an incentive for a struggling new nurse saddled with college loans. Duke University Hospital instituted a retention bonus system for four distinct positions that balances tenure with a graduated bonus. According to J. Robert Clapp, Jr. (2002), chief operating officer at Duke University Hospital, each employee is offered a retention bonus if they complete three years of service from a particular date. The amount of the bonus is based on length of time the individual has been with the hospital. For example, in hypothetical dollars, the bonus for a 15-year employee may be $7,500 in three years, while the bonus for a 10-year employee may come to $5,000 in three years. Since this bonus was introduced in 2001, Duke University Hospital has experienced a dramatic improvement in turnover among pharmacists, respiratory therapists, and radiology technicians. A modest turnover improvement among nurses has also been observed since the inception of the system.

Another retention bonus is affectionately known as "golden handcuffs." It typically bestows significant financial gain, either directly or indirectly, to the recipient. Such gain comes with conditions of employment and creates financial loss if the employee leaves the company. A common example is the leased-car bonus. Companies frequently lease a car for members of the sales team, actually putting the lease in the individual's name. If the sales rep stays with the company, the lease is paid for by the employer. If the individual leaves, the unpaid portion of the lease becomes his or her own responsibility. The same principle applies to tuition reimbursement for educational courses at a college or university.

Tuition is paid as long as the employee remains with the company. However, if employment is terminated, the individual is responsible for the remaining tuition. This clearly creates an economic incentive to stay. In some cases, companies also require employees to continue their employment for a specified period of time following graduation so that they can reap the benefits of the education. If the employee chooses to leave, he or she must repay a portion of the tuition to the organization. Sometimes, however, no continued-employment strings are attached to educational support. For example, Johnson & Johnson and AstraZeneca do not require employees to stay for a predetermined length of time to take advantage of tuition reimbursement. Their 'brand" serves as a powerful draw. Educational commitment to employees without strings is merely a component of the brand.

Healthcare organizations have also implemented golden handcuff bonuses. During the Y2K-preparedness crisis in the late 1990s, one healthcare system offered golden handcuffs to their information technology (IT) staff to maximize retention. A retention differential ranging from 5 percent to 20 percent of base salary was offered to each regular full-time IT employee. On top of that, a bonus was paid for continued employment, which also ranged from 5 percent to 20 percent of base salary. This resulted in zero turnover, the original intended effect. However, in retrospect, this initiative was considered overkill by its designers in that an excessive amount of money was spent to achieve a favorable result that insiders believe probably would have occurred without the additional $5 million expense. More important, however, was that the bonus created an entitlement mentality among the IT group. As a result, it has been difficult to wean IT workers from expectations of unusually generous paychecks. Perhaps most important was the understanding of the issue of turnover itself. Some turnover is actually healthy for an organization, especially when the infusion of new ideas is desirable, although ensuring retention during a critical time period may be deemed most important.

Bonuses are also offered to employees who refer prospective candidates for hire. Companies value these referrals because candidates are prescreened to some degree by the worker already employed by the organization, which saves valuable recruiting time and money. There are also advantages on the post-hire side as well. If the candidate is hired, knowing someone in the new company may ease his or her transition into the organization. This practice, already employed to some extent in hospitals, is used frequently in other industries. Of *Fortune*'s 100 Best Companies to Work For in 2001, 83 paid employees a bonus for a successful new hire referral (*Fortune* 2001). The amounts can be substantial. Deloitte & Touche, another company on both the *Fortune*'s and *Working Mother*'s lists, paid up to $15,000 for each successful referral. University of Maryland Medical Center offers employee-referral bonuses for high-impact and difficult-to-recruit areas. The amounts vary between $500 and $3,000 depending on the position referred, and subsequent referrals are paid at a higher rate to encourage repeat referrals. The bonuses are paid to the referring employee once the new hire completes 18 months of employment. Miami Valley Hospital pays employees $1,000 bonuses for referrals who are hired and complete a 90-day probationary period.

Although there is no defined return on investment in the literature for employee referral bonuses, general consensus suggests that the practice does pay off substantially. "Prescreened applicants" come to work with at least a loose alliance with the corporate culture through the referring employee. Because the company typically pays a fee to an outside placement agency, the practice of employee referrals saves money. For some companies, a portion of these savings gets redirected to a bonus for a current employee. Typically, these employee-referral bonus programs pay at varying rates depending on referred position. Management positions frequently command higher bonus dollars than front-line staff positions. But not everyone is eligible to participate in the program. At some companies, employees eligible for referral bonuses must be below a certain level and not in the direct chain of management of the person to be hired. In other organizations, human resources staff members are ineligible because recruiting is one of their primary responsibilities. Perhaps most significant to note is the preferential treatment these job candidates get. At many companies, preference is given to employee-referred applicants before outside applicants, assuming all things are equal. In organizations where there are 2,000 to 3,000 applicants for each position, employee referrals saves managers considerable time; managers evaluate employee referrals prior to those coming from the outside. In the best-designed programs, effective controls are built into the process. Employees need to be discriminating in their referrals given that bonuses are typically only awarded after their referral has been hired and retained for at least six months.

Just how effective are employee-referral bonuses? Consensus suggests that they are highly effective. As a result, this approach is used extensively across industries, including healthcare. The Dallas-Fort Worth Hospital Council, which lists recruitment and retention as one of its top concerns, reported that employee-referral programs are more effective than signing bonuses in recruiting new workers (*The Dallas Morning News* 2000). The practice was used extensively in the technology industry during the late 1990s and into 2000. Fifty percent of the new hires in 2000 at LSI Logic Corporation— a company in Milpitas, California, that produces semiconductors—came from employee referrals (*San Jose Mercury News* 2000). At CISCO, which hired on average between 1,800 and 2,000 people each quarter in 1999, an estimated 40 percent to 60 percent of new hires came from employee referrals (*Chicago Tribune* 1999). According to Barbara Smith (2002), 50 percent of applicants at Miami Valley Hospital were referrals from employees.

Strategy 3: Leveraging Formal Recognition Programs

Much like companies in other industries, hospitals employ formal recognition programs to increase employee satisfaction. Interest in recognition programs stems at least in part from the role a positive work climate plays in job satisfaction and retention. Recognition programs make up one piece of that positive work climate. Exactly what comprises recognition programs is almost as varied as the companies themselves.

Customer service awards, employee tenure awards, trips, cash, celebration banquets, and other gifts are just some examples of recognition that rewards performance. Toyota Manufacturing USA spends about $250,000 annually on a "perfect-attendance" meeting for high-attendance employees. The prior day's accomplishments are broadcast in daily teleconference meetings at FedEx Corporation as a way of recognizing individuals who achieved desired business results. At CISCO, the CEO holds a monthly "birthday breakfast" meeting for anyone with a recent birthday. During this meeting, the CEO answers every question he is asked. To prevent employees from feeling inhibited about asking controversial questions, CISCO discourages directors and vice presidents from attending the meetings. At CISCO, recognition rewards are *expected* to be offered. In fact, any CISCO employee can give anybody else a recognition reward ranging from a free dinner to a $5,000 check, with the approval of the employee's manager. Performance management systems ensure that this practice occurs. Supervisors' performance appraisals include a measure on whether their reward budgets were spent.

Some companies also hold events to recognize their employees and encourage a sense of community. Ben & Jerry's Homemade Ice Cream has a "joy gang" that organizes such events as Cajun parties, ping pong tournaments, and manufacturing appreciation days. CISCO holds Christmas parties that feature 100 food stations and entertainment, including Elvis imitators. Valassis Company, a company that produces newspaper inserts in Livonia, Michigan, and one of *Fortune's* 100 Best Companies to Work For in 2001 and 2002, rented an airplane hangar and offered airplane rides to all who attended. This organization experienced only 7 percent turnover in 1999 (*Fortune* 2001). A recognition initiative used at Bank of America is called the CELA, the Customer Experience Leadership Award. A CELA is a display plaque that signifies recognition of good performance. Anyone can give a CELA to anyone else within the organization. For example, if a customer writes a positive letter about an associate, the associate's manager might present him or her a CELA in recognition of the service that led to the letter. But granting a CELA is not limited to managers; associates can present them as well. At the end of the year, managers submit names to human resources based on the number and type of CELAs received. The human resources department then distributes larger monetary awards to a subset of that group in a formal recognition ceremony. Then, an elite subset of that group is selected to become part of the "Dream Team." This small group is rewarded with abundant recognition, culminating in a trip to a desirable locale such as New Orleans. Again, this program is promoted extensively throughout the organization, rewarding behavior that is consistent with corporate goals.

Miami Valley Hospital (MVH) provides a best-practice example of employee recognition in a hospital setting. MVH uses several approaches to recognize individuals. They give out traditional service awards in the form of gift certificates to employees for three, five, and ten years of service and for every five years of service after that. Annual banquets honor employees who have reached 10 and 15 years of tenure. At 20 years of service, an individual is inducted into the 20-Year Club and given lifetime membership. An annual banquet that is attended by over 1,000 people, including current staff and retirees, is held for these individuals. Other recognition initiatives include quarterly events held in the cafeteria for all employees based on varying themes, a Wall of Excellence that posts employees who demonstrated exemplary customer service, and letters from the president that go out approximately three times per year thanking employees for their contributions. Gift certificates add to the appreciation. Although all of these programs are important for retention, Barbara Smith (2002), MVH's director of human resources, notes that the most significant and powerful recognition comes from immediate supervisors who acknowledge the contributions of their direct reports. In light of MVH's commitment to this principle, all managers get feedback on the effectiveness of their practices in this and related areas. They are held accountable for effective performance through management bonuses and performance review.

Through their Corporate University, Baptist Health Care conducts a survey on staff recognition that provides a record of what individuals prefer for their own reward and recognition. Employees rank types of recognition on a scale, which then provides information on how to personalize recognition for individuals in a way that will have the most impact on them. For example, while some individuals may prefer a quiet pat on the back for a job well done and a small token of appreciation, others may seek public acknowledgement of their accomplishment in a staff meeting or a companywide newsletter. This survey enables managers to customize recognition, promoting employee satisfaction and retention.

In today's economy, marked by recessionary conditions, organizations are under pressure to dispense with recognition programs to cut expenses. Although some companies have cut back on the rewards and some eliminated programs altogether, most continue with the basic structure. These companies recognize the importance of creating a positive workplace for employees to promote retention long term. In healthcare, which is not as vulnerable to economic fluctuations as other industries, it is crucial that organizations continue their effective recognition programs to retain those workers they have strived so hard to recruit and keep.

Strategy 4: Implementing Active Communication Programs

Aggressive communication programs have proven to have beneficial effects on employee turnover. Based on NAI's research, there is empirical evidence that pursuing such a communication strategy as a supplement to effective management practices results in lower employee absenteeism, reduced turnover, and higher productivity. But this strategy alone doesn't work, as one healthcare organization sadly discovered.

Executives at one large Midwestern not-for-profit hospital hoped to increase morale and decrease turnover by publishing more information for the benefit of staff. Although engaging in broad communications appeared to be a worthwhile use of resources, it was not. Committed to trying to improve the quality of information exchanged throughout the institution, the hospital's senior administration orchestrated large-scale forums, committing resources to building town-hall-type meetings and more "broadcast" style communications. At the same time they failed to appreciate the role of the first-line manager in building identification with the organization as well as in carrying "official" messages up, down, and across the hierarchy. Results on a subsequent employee work-climate survey were quite disappointing. Scores jumped dramatically regarding senior management's "interest" in employees, but they remained marginal as before regarding senior management's perceived "response" to concerns. The resulting disparity in perception only widened the existing credibility gap and further undermined employee identification with the organization. The implicit message was clear: Don't get my expectation up (i.e., ask my opinion) if you're not going to do anything about it.

The moral of the example is that communication programs must be enhanced in conjunction with other retention mechanisms and infrastructure supports (e.g., management effectiveness and changes to core business process) to be successful.

Despite this unfortunate example, a number of mechanisms are very effective in promoting communication within organizations that result in significant positive performance shifts when linked to line efforts. Some companies hold meetings for all employees at regular intervals to communicate the strategy of the company and to ensure all employees feel included. At Allstate Insurance Company, agents meet with executives three times per year at forums to cement that identification. CISCO holds quarterly "all hands" meetings to communicate high-level strategies and keep everyone in the loop. CISCO also provides webcasts of important events, delivering information right to employees' desktops. Saturn assemblers receive information continuously through their internal television network. Security Benefit Group in Topeka, Kansas, announces financial information at quarterly all-associates meetings to ensure that everyone is aware of how the company is performing. Duke University Hospital uses strategically placed video monitors to highlight important breaking news. In all of these cases the broadcast messages are built on a foundation of effective dialog at the local managerial level. Expectations of managers are very clear. They, in turn, must discuss the implications of the broadcast with their staff at local meetings.

At Miami Valley Hospital a formal communication vehicle is in place to ensure employees are kept in the loop and that senior management receives appropriate information through direct access. Approximately three times per month, the president and/or chief operating officer meets with a group of 15 or so employees for breakfast, lunch, or dinner. These individuals are selected by their managers if they want to participate; the goal is for everyone to get a turn. During these meetings, the president or COO conveys information and then gives employees a chance to ask questions. According to Barbara Smith (2002), people are quite candid during these discussions, providing good dialog and surfacing important concerns. What is most important, however, is the follow-up to issues raised to ensure that concerns are addressed, whether at that meeting or in subsequent discussions.

Clearly, feedback is just as important for communication as broadcasting. Without it, employees are likely to feel that their concerns are being ignored. This critical component of communicating can be accomplished in a couple of different ways. A substantial percentage of organizations conduct employee surveys, as discussed extensively in Chapter 4. The same principles regarding surveys hold true in other industries as in healthcare. The most significant point noted earlier is that employees perceive the value in the survey by observing changes that occur based on survey results. In addition, surveys serve as a valuable management tool by providing benchmark satisfaction data and giving insight into future retention. If done robustly, employee climate surveys also assess the impact and ultimate effectiveness of management and organizational practices.

Another option for receiving feedback is to initiate a hotline. At Allstate, agents access a confidential, toll-free resolution line to express their problems and receive support. Employees at Toyota can access their hotline number from any phone. Human resources reviews and investigates all of the messages received. If the call is anonymous, the questions and Toyota's response are posted on plant bulletin boards. If not anonymous, the caller receives a personal response. Healthcare organizations often use hotlines as well, as reflected in our top-100 hospital survey results. Miami Valley Hospital instituted a president's hotline in 1988. According to its president, Bill Thornton, all callers are contacted within 24 hours, receiving a letter directly from him. If a specific area, such as human resources, is identified as problematic, an investigation will occur and a second letter will be sent by the president on resolution of the matter. This hotline is used extensively by employees and by anyone else with a concern. It has proven to be an effective method for identifying employee concerns and addressing them before they become significant issues. In summary, it cannot be overemphasized that excellent communications play a critical role in successful management. But like bonus programs and recognition, communication must be carefully structured and be built on a solid base of managerial accountability.

Strategy 5: Aligning Hiring and Orientation Strategies with Retention Strategies

A basic strategy frequently employed by organizations in other industries is to match hiring strategies with retention strategies. For example, organizations that are serious about service bring in candidates who are committed to strong service orientations. Ritz Carlton, Southwest Airlines, Disney, and Nordstrom's are but a few companies noted for this type of alignment. Even organizations bombarded with high-volume hiring targets to meet corporate growth goals understand the importance of the match. By aligning hiring strategies with retention, productivity gains and employee retention are more likely.

One such strategy involves communicating promotional opportunities *and* the corporate culture to applicants so that both parties have sufficient information to decide if they provide the right fit for each other. Carrying this concept further, a current employee may be asked to interact with the applicant during non-working hours to create a personal bond, answer any questions, and get a better sense of fit. Both parties, the applicant and organization, are seeking congruity so that there is a higher probability that the relationship will be long term. Although the up-front costs in time are significant, these investments may be offset down the road by reduced turnover costs.

At the base of this activity is the belief that applicants should align with the basic values of the organization. By using value-based hiring screens, candidates will be selected if their values match those of the company. Clearly, hiring the right people who emulate the organization's ideology and meet competency requirements saves money in the long run. For example, Ben & Jerry's Homemade Ice Cream screens out candidates who aren't committed to the firm's social goals of environmental conservation. Goldman Sachs Group, a financial services company, looks for prospective employees who emphasize integrity, value autonomy, and can work in a fluid and changing structure. Toyota conducts an extensive five-day testing and interviewing program that focuses on teamwork, among other attributes.

Although recruiting to achieve the right fit saves considerable dollars in turnover costs, many organizations complain about the time, effort, and money spent sorting through stacks of job applications. However, at Southwest Airlines, where they received 200,000 applications for 5,000 openings in 1999, leaders don't feel that sifting through the paper is a waste of time (*Trustee* 2000). Instead, they recognize the importance of hiring the right people who will lead them to continued success as an organization. Once an employee has been hired, organizations in other industries go to great lengths to ensure that the orientation period is as smooth as possible. In one IT company, integration teams mobilize to ensure that the new employee is set up on the intranet, has an office space that is in optimal working order, and has access to supplies. A formal orientation is scheduled and managers must adhere to defined milestones in providing a departmental orientation. Peers assigned to each new hire provide other information and assist with the indoctrination into the company.

CISCO's Fast Start program notifies a facility team when a new employee is hired. The facility team ensures that the new employee has a completely functional workspace, has an assigned peer within the company to answer questions, and is enrolled in a two-day orientation course.

The best companies build an extensive orientation program for new employees to help acculturate them and learn the company's products and services. Orientation for new managers—whether new to the company or merely new to management within the company—is also critical in ensuring alignment. For example, Security Benefit Group (SBG) provides an SBG Management Fundamentals program that introduces managers to the core SBG values and managers' own role in living them and ensuring that others do as well. Some of the top-100 hospitals in our survey have begun to adopt this approach. Duke University Hospital has instituted a similar approach called "Managing at Duke." With acculturation clearly as a focal intent, Miami Valley Hospital has made new employee orientation an opportunity to enhance the acculturation process.

Strategy 6: Ensuring Managerial Effectiveness and Accountability for Retention

Throughout this book we have argued that the most important determinant of employee satisfaction is the extent to which a hospital has put in place effective management practices. In addition, the proper management infrastructure, including appropriate spans of control, must be in place to enable managers to achieve optimal efficiencies and effectiveness in leading their staff. As experience has shown across industries, employees must interact frequently with their managers. The quality of this contact is what has the greatest impact on the employee's propensity to stay or leave an organization. Well-developed managers who are capable of managing complex processes and gaining rapid insight into employee issues to resolve them will have maximum positive impact on retention.

As we discussed in Chapter 5, managers need to be held accountable for turnover within their spans of control. Managers in other industries, where retention is tracked on a more regular basis, are called on the carpet for excessive turnover. Results may be reflected in performance appraisals as issues are identified and handled. For example, at one banking institution, managerial bonuses are linked to maintaining the 97 percent retention rate that is in place. Although 97 percent retention is a laudable goal, we recognize that this figure is unrealistic for most organizations and may not provide the necessary turnover required to infuse new ideas into the company. A more optimal turnover rate may be 6 percent to 10 percent, depending on the industry. Because job replacement is a costly proposition, an organization cannot afford to tolerate excessive turnover.

Clearly, managers must be held accountable for the complex operational aspects of their organization—that is, for financial management, quality outcomes, employee satisfaction that provides a direct and key link to patient satisfaction, and customer/patient satisfaction. All of these performance factors relate to employee retention. As one major healthcare institution found, by emphasizing managerial accountability and the performance of their "small business," they reduced their turnover rate from 19 percent to 6 percent. This was attributed to deliberate attention to building identification with strategic business goals, clarity of performance expectations, team cohesiveness within units, creation of the "right" environment, and promoting respect for nurses from physicians—a common issue in hospitals.

In other industries, as well as in selected healthcare organizations, mechanisms have been developed to ensure management accountability for program performance and for retention. For many years, FedEx has made a commitment to accountability for key performance indicators, one of which is to track on-time delivery. On a daily basis, managers and staff meet to review those packages that were not delivered within acceptable time frame and quality standards. The data drive improvements in systems and guide managers to address substandard performance. Building a standard of excellence that drives continued performance improvement is a source of pride for most employees, especially those who have been carefully screened for such a fit.

Another shining example in healthcare where management accountability is emphasized is at Miami Valley Hospital. The executive management team there looks to all employees (managerial and nonmanagerial) to report where the hospital has vulnerabilities, to identify what types of issues exist, and to suggest what appropriate solutions should be taken. So every three years since 1988, the organization conducts a comprehensive organizational practices survey of all its employees to identify strengths and areas that need improvement. To respond effectively to survey results, managers must develop action plans to correct those areas identified, engaging further employee input to clarify and amplify the issues. These action plans are monitored by executive management, who holds those responsible accountable for the improvements. Mini-surveys are also conducted on an annual basis to track progress on these issues and identify whether improvements are resulting in better survey scores. To drive accountability further, merit reviews for vice presidents and directors are structured to include increases based on survey results. In addition, vice presidents can link action plans for areas of improvement to managerial merit increases, providing a financial incentive for effective improvements.

Edward Case (2002), the chief executive officer at Presbyterian Healthcare in Charlotte, North Carolina, strongly believes that employees look to their supervisor for support. Within his organization, not unlike other healthcare institutions, clinical managers are traditionally promoted on their clinical abilities, not on their managerial abilities. To measure managerial competence, the hospital conducts a survey semiannually that focuses on employees' assessment of their direct managers at all levels. The results of this survey provide areas of emphasis and focus for the education department in determining management-development needs. One of the main components of the survey is communication. According to Case, "Managers recognize that the more time they communicate and are visible, the more successful they will be [in retention results]." Trends across time are also examined, and results are analyzed through the entire reporting chain to observe the cascading effect of positive communication or to identify levels of weakness within the organizational structure. According to Case, managers understand that this is a very serious situation and that action will be taken based on survey results. Not surprisingly, the managers with the highest scores have the best retention rates. Presbyterian Healthcare also promotes retention by going to great lengths to be flexible and responsive to employee situations. They will accommodate the diversity of their employee needs by enabling scheduling flexibility within acceptable parameters.

Security Benefit Group also conducts organizational practices surveys to identify vulnerabilities in management behavior. If scores are low on a consistent basis for a particular manager, they will use the tool to support employment-related decisions. For example, management incentives (and disincentives) may be linked to survey results. If a particular manager has consistently higher negative turnover than his or her counterparts, his or her individual management incentive plan will be linked to future turnover results. To support stronger performance, the manager will receive individualized training in areas identified as vulnerable on the survey. In addition, performance evaluations linking back to organizational goals are required and used actively throughout the year for all managers.

Yale-New Haven Hospital in Connecticut has also been actively engaged in ensuring managerial effectiveness. In the early 1990s the hospital underwent restructuring and cost cutting that resulted in significantly reduced staff and increased spans of control. The fallout from these changes included decreased employee satisfaction and associated problems. So in 1998, the hospital began a process to revisit its management roles and responsibilities. Through this process, the organization developed job charters for its patient care manager roles, which included key accountabilities for the position, key interfaces and responsibilities, and decision-making authority. Next were the creation of defined competencies necessary to be successful in this position and the development of training and systems to support these competencies. As a result of this powerful process, patient care managers have realized they're an integral part in the success of organizational change. Outcomes have included a decrease in the number of patient complaints regarding attention of assigned caregivers and other improvements in areas such as financial performance, patient satisfaction, and physician satisfaction. Along with the positive movement in these directions, employee turnover also began to decline. With infrastructure modifications in place to support managerial effectiveness, patient care managers could effect positive change to improve the organizational environment.

Strategy 7: Partnering with Training or Teaching Organizations

Partnering with an educational organization creates a labor pool from a specific source, if the organization agrees to preferential hiring from that source. For example, a hospital in partnership with a university has input into the school's curriculum design, ensuring that it provides skills and competencies required by the hospital. As a result, both sides win. After graduation, students are given first priority in employment with the partner hospital. The hospital recommends future students to the program based on the perceived quality and relevance of the curriculum. Other options include internships, where the student works at the organization to get "hands on" experience while in school and will then be eligible for employment with the organization after graduation. This arrangement also enables these potential candidates to become familiar with the organization during employment, resulting in their need for less training. More forward-looking hospitals, including Yale-New Haven Hospital, have focused on the quality of the students' experience to ensure that students want to return as employees.

The U.S. Army has a program called "Partnership for Youth Services," or PaYS, that facilitates partnerships between select companies and the Army. The program brings significant advantage to partner companies. Essentially, the Army assumes training responsibility for the company's future employees in agreed-on skill areas. Employment is guaranteed once the service term in the Army is complete. To be eligible for the program, individuals must commit to working for a particular member employer. Once committed, the Army provides training in the requisite skills. Six months prior to separation from the Army, participating individuals begin their transition to civilian life and to the company preselected as an employer. Final coordination with the company, including application, interviews, and preemployment visits, occurs prior to leaving the Army. This program provides employers with qualified individuals available for employment at agreed-on timeframes. Such "feeder" programs have existed in healthcare for years. University-based hospitals, for example, have built-in advantages if they can hire students from their associated college or university. These students usually conduct their internships or practicums at the hospital, providing real work output while learning the structure (and culture) of the hospital environment. Because the student becomes accustomed to the particular hospital, he or she will more likely seek employment in the familiar environment, assuming the experience was positive. This results in a win-win proposition for everyone, developing the skills of the healthcare worker while luring new talent for the hospital.

Yale-New Haven Hospital has initiated an extensive plan to address these partnering relationships. The first step in their process is to identify nursing schools that provide exceptional training and then develop a relationship with them. Next, specific initiatives are implemented with individual schools, including the design and development of a collaborative two-year nursing program and establishment of clinical work-study programs. The latter initiative develops nursing student competencies and provides preferred placement status for participants. Yale-New Haven Hospital has also expanded partnerships with existing educational collaborators to provide student clinical assistants and student nurse assistants. To facilitate the educational component of these programs, the hospital expanded the Clinical Teaching Partnership program to support and develop both its nurse preceptors and students. To capitalize on its educational efforts, the hospital also developed a preferred hiring program for new graduates who have worked at the hospital as student clinical assistants and student nurse assistants. These alliances provide Yale-New Haven Hospital an additional recruitment stream of prospective employees who are more likely to have the requisite skills needed to be successful at that hospital.

Even though it is a community and not a university teaching hospital, Miami Valley Hospital has strong relationships with the nursing schools in the Dayton, Ohio area. At one time, the hospital had its own nursing school; when the school closed, students were absorbed into other institutions. However, the hospital's relationship with these other institutions remained strong. Miami Valley Hospital's continued focus on new graduates and nursing students has been key to its success. The hospital actively recruits nursing students to work as patient care technicians. It has also developed an Extern Program for junior-level and senior-level nursing students that offers internships and hence an expanded relationship with the organization that can lead to preferential hiring.

In all of these examples this key point stands out: Successful recruitment streams require (1) commitment to new grads and the institutions that teach them and (2) an internal hospital culture to attract and nurture them.

Strategy 8: Adopting Aggressive Development

Development and training opportunities not only attract employees to an organization, they also retain workers who value developmental opportunities. Many avenues for employee development exist, and companies must be cognizant of the options available. Generally, the greater the investment in training, the higher the probability of achieving goals. The airline industry provides a great example. At Singapore Airlines, 15 percent of the payroll goes into employee training, versus 1.5 percent for U.S. airlines (*Trustee* 2000). To highlight this further, Singapore Airline's flight attendants' formal training program lasts for four months, versus the four weeks standard for U.S. airlines. This attention to training has paid off for the airline in terms of awards. Singapore Airlines was the top airline cited in *Fortune*'s list of World's Most Admired Companies. It has also garnered customer service awards, including Best Overall Airline from the Business Traveler Awards, and was named the best international carrier for the 13th time in 14 years by *Conde Nast Traveler* in 2001. Clearly, this is an example of training that has a bottom-line impact!

Johnson & Johnson, IBM, Motorola, Disney, and AstraZeneca represent other examples of companies that have long recognized the need for extensive and ongoing individual and managerial development. Continued learning is an expectation in each of these organizations and extensive programs are in place to meet the developmental needs of employees annually, including the support of in-house training and development organizations. More senior managers are also held accountable to ensure that development plans that are created are implemented. Typically for these organizations, the development plans form the basis of succession-planning efforts.

Development may also be targeted toward high-potential performers. Best-in-class organizations make significant investments in the development of such employees, as we'll discuss later in this chapter. Along with strong emphasis on developmental assignments and training, increased compensation and benefit packages paid out over a period of time complete the package.

For most organizations, however, the primary mode of employee development entails some form of on-the-job training (OJT). This activity is crucial in getting new employees up to speed; thus, it affects ultimate job success. Failing to adequately structure this experience, or eliminating it with across-the-board budget cuts, will undermine quality and retention. Design of OJT may be formal, with a defined curriculum, or may be informal, which is more frequently the case across industries. Regardless of the type of OJT, all content areas must be covered in a timely fashion so that new staff members have sufficient information to perform their responsibilities independently as intended.

At best organizations, managers take employee training quite seriously and devote extensive resources toward effective employee performance. One example brings this alive. At Security Benefit Group, an extensive organizational practices survey identified the need for improvement in customer satisfaction with one of their call centers. The survey showed that employees in this area required stronger relationship-management skills in dealing with their customers. To address this need, SBG developed a comprehensive training module on managing relationships for all employees in this department. This has had successful results, and it provides needed linkage between associate development and customer satisfaction, a critical success factor for the organization.

Baptist Health Care has "Corporate University" in which about 550 leaders and managers participate in the leadership development program, which involves off-site day-long training on a quarterly basis. Every individual who participates in this program must demonstrate results from a process called "Cascade Training." According to Pam Bilbrey (2002), senior vice president of corporate development at Baptist Health Care, every participant in Corporate University must take the materials from their course (which may include slides, manuals, scripts, exercises, surveys, and various handouts) and then teach the concepts to their own staff. Included in the Cascade Training kit is a Leader's Accountability form that records this transfer of knowledge. Corporate development then compiles and monitors the results and reports compliance to the vice president. The hospital planned to initiate two more programs through the Corporate University in 2002 and 2003 entitled "College for Performance Excellence" and "College for Clinical Excellence." Both programs will link training to the core strategies for the organization.

At Duke University Hospital, all middle managers go through a curriculum called "Managing at Duke." This program was developed in response to the results of a value-driven survey, which showed that employees felt their manager was the most crucial factor in satisfaction with their jobs, a result that is congruent with the principles cited in this book. According to J. Robert Clapp, Jr. (2002), chief operating officer at Duke University Hospital, this three-day program held at the Duke University Business School provides a value-based approach to training for what's important to staff and ties these values into what's important at Duke. The curriculum provides training in the core competencies for managers, and then it tailors these competencies to the way things work at Duke. Follow-up to Managing at Duke occurs several ways: (1) supervisors of attendees complete assessments post-course to evaluate the impact on the managers; (2) attendees become members of an alumni association, which is brought together as a group post-course to modify the curriculum for future sessions; (3) there is public recognition of the participants; and (4) the attendees are used to test new concepts for hospital initiatives.

Tuition reimbursement for ongoing educational training has also been a popular retention tool, but it has been curtailed to some degree recently by flat economic conditions that affect what many regard as discretionary company spending. Typically, companies pay all or a portion of the cost of tuition. Frequently, reimbursement depends on a "screen" of applicability to the job, future promotion, or grades received. At Intermec Corporation, a high-tech data-collection company in Everett, Washington, tuition for approved coursework is reimbursed at 100 percent and books are reimbursed at 50 percent. As mentioned earlier in this chapter, some companies require employees who receive tuition reimbursement to stay with the organization for a designated period of time after graduation. If not, these employees must repay a portion of the tuition. One notable exception is Johnson & Johnson, a leading company that is on a multitude of "best" lists and does not have this requirement. AstraZeneca, a leading pharmaceutical company, also does not have this requirement for their generous tuition reimbursement policy. AstraZeneca pays up to 100 percent of the costs of tuition, books, and entrance exams, depending on the employee's status. The company's general maximum contribution is $10,000 per year, but this can be exceeded based on circumstances. There are also scholarships available for family members of employees, according to Teresa Bien (2002), director of medical affairs-training at AstraZeneca. In addition, the company sponsors full tuition for a select group of individuals to receive their executive M.B.A., Ph.D., and J.D. degrees.

Tuition reimbursement is a natural extension of benefits for university-based hospital systems. In recognition of the needs of its employees, the University of Maryland Medical Center (UMMC) enhanced tuition benefits for its staff as an approach to promote retention and to stimulate recruitment. UMMC took this one step further. It now offers tuition assistance for dependents of many clinical employees in the amount of up to $10,000 per child. This action enables UMMC to remain competitive with Johns Hopkins Hospital, another major medical employer in the area. Johns Hopkins also provides up to 100 percent tuition reimbursement for staff and 50 percent tuition assistance for dependents. This policy has been met with favorable reactions at UMMC.

With an experienced in-house training department, particular competencies can be developed, legally mandated education can be offered, and technical skills can be enhanced so that employees can be more successful in their jobs. Like most hospitals in the top 100, Intermec Corporation's training department offers courses in performance management, conducting legal interviews, business writing, and influence strategies for managers. Saturn, the automobile manufacturer, holds a career-growth workshop that uses vocational guidance tools to help employees identify skills they need to develop.

Other options for training exist. Seminars and special programs sponsored by third parties to teach critical-skills development occur frequently and may be brought in-house. In addition, conferences offer continuing education credits and opportunities for networking and are often funded by companies. Hospitals also recognize the criticality of providing ongoing education beyond mandatory education. Many hospitals make concerted efforts to recognize the value of continuing education, offering limited funds to support continuing education for each employee annually. Other industries have placed great emphasis on development for a number of years. Within the medical affairs department at AstraZeneca, every staff member is allocated $4,000 per year in professional development costs. This is in addition to full sponsorship of membership in two professional associations per year and payment of all professional licensures. Clearly, development matters.

Even educational systems increasingly recognize the business impact of employee development. Nevada's Clark County School District, which includes Las Vegas, has initiated a new teacher welcoming center, networking and mentoring program, and more extended training. The results have been striking. Ninety-six percent of new teachers remained after their first year, compared to only about 60 percent in other districts (*Philadelphia Inquirer* 2001). In summary, development will facilitate employee retention. It has become an expected activity by many employees and seen as table stakes for employers.

Strategy 9: Providing Family-Friendly Benefits and Policies

Various other inducements create an environment that is conducive to employee retention. Many of these address a growing area of concern to employees: the extent to which employers are "family friendly." The degree to which organizational policies and practices support an employee's family life may actually influence the employee's decision to join a company and may affect the decision to stay. More than ever before, companies are realizing the impact of job stress on family life and health. Consider that 51 percent of families with children have two working parents, which is a 54 percent increase over 1977 figures (*Working Mother* 2001). On top of this, full-time workers on average work more hours today than they did 20 years ago, an additional source of stress that puts pressure on work-life balance. In response, organizations are redesigning the structure of work policies where possible to reduce job-related stress. One bank, in recognition of work-life balance, actually requires employees to commit to three business goals and three personal goals in their performance development plans. Managers are held accountable for ensuring that their staff meet their personal and business goals.

Some innovative companies have tried to reduce stress by helping their employees manage the logistics of their lives, actions that harken back to the "company towns" prevalent during the first part of the last century. CISCO, for example, provides on-site stores, dry cleaning services, ATMs, automobile oil changes, fitness centers, and mobile dental clinics for their employees. Unlike most large employers, CISCO encourages employees to be "CISCO centric," having most of their needs attended to at their workplace. In one of the less typical categories, Computer Associates offers its employees financial assistance to buy homes near its headquarters in New York.

Numerous policies and benefits fall into the family-friendly category. One of the most significant examples involves support for child care. In many organizations, on-site day care provides convenience for working parents. Security Benefit Group, for example, provides a day care center called "SBG Academy." This facility is the cornerstone of the family-friendly benefits policy at SBG, according to Craig Anderson (2002), senior vice president of human resources. Merck & Co., a pharmaceutical company, has four on-site child care centers in New Jersey and Pennsylvania with a capacity of 900 children. With higher-than-typical caregiver-to-child ratios and expanded hours, Merck subsidizes almost 20 percent of the cost. The company's reward for its efforts is a mere 9 percent voluntary turnover rate in 1999 and 10 percent in 2000. Merck appears on both *Fortune's* and *Working Mother's* 100 Best Companies lists. Some companies offer day care subsidies, while others design programs in which day care expenses are tax exempt. This latter example, managed under government-allowed "Flexible Spending Accounts," also covers medical expenses. To be eligible, employers merely must follow the rules dictated by the IRS in administering the plans.

Other family-friendly benefits include generous maternity or paternity leaves (e.g., six to twelve months) or leaves to care for an ill family member. State and federal regulations provide for this leave under the Family Leave and Medical Act, but requirements only apply to companies with a minimum number of employees. Bank of America, which has been on *Working Mother's* 100 Best Companies list for three years, offers new mothers two fully paid weeks of maternity leave for each year of service, job-guaranteed paternity leave up to 26 weeks for new fathers, and paid leave for adoptive parents and foster caregivers. Goldman Sachs Group, which appears on both *Working Mother's* and *Fortune's* 100 Best Companies lists (number 15 in 2001 and number 19 in 2002) offers a standard 16-week, full-pay maternity leave. In addition to this they have an Infant Transition Program, which allows babies up to six months old to spend 40 days in an on-site child care center. Like many East Coast companies, the New York-based firm provided counseling to its own employees following the attacks on the World Trade Center on September 11,

2001. MBNA America Bank, listed among both *Fortune*'s and *Working Mother*'s 100 Best Companies, provides a 24-hour hotline for medical advice and provides up to $20,000 in support for adoption. In many other organizations, leaves are also available for adoptions.

Employee assistance programs (EAPs) are often provided by employers at little or no charge. Originally evolving from programs by Eastman Kodak Company and E.I. du Pont in the 1940s that treat alcoholism, EAPs now assist individuals by providing resources, referral, or counseling services or any combination of the three. McDonald's Corporation offers a national McResource Line, a resource and referral service that provides counseling and help with child care and elder issues for a nominal fee to employees. Accountants for Ernst & Young, LLP work vigorously during the tax season of January through April. To alleviate the accumulated stress, accountants are rewarded with paid and sometimes nonpaid summer sabbaticals for four to eight weeks. Even though Ernst & Young appears on both *Fortune*'s and *Working Mother*'s 100 Best Companies lists, the company experienced high turnover in 1999 and 2000—that is, 28 percent and 26 percent respectively. This suggests one critical lesson: All the family-friendly policies in the world may not contain turnover, depending on other factors at work.

Flexible work arrangements is an increasingly popular family-friendly policy. Covering myriad options, flexible work arrangements facilitate work-life balance. One common example is flextime, which allows employees to adjust work start and stop times. Used prevalently throughout a variety of industries, flextime has little impact on the volume or quality of actual work accomplished, as long as employees are available for work during "critical" portions of the day and for planned meeting times. Compressed work weeks are another common option. With compressed work weeks, employees work the total number of required hours in a given week but do it within a shorter period of time. For example, if 40 hours is the standard work week within a company, an employee can choose to work Monday through Thursday for ten hours a day rather than the traditional Monday through Friday for eight hours a day. In companies where this work structure is in effect, the same caveat applies to this arrangement as with flextime: Employees must be available during critical portions of the work week.

Bristol-Myers Squibb, a pharmaceutical company ranked by *Working Mothers* as one of the ten best companies, formalized a flex program in 2000. As a result, by the end of 2000, 8 percent of the company's 22,000 U.S. employees were using compressed work weeks, job sharing, telecommuting, flextime, or part-time arrangements. First Tennessee Bank, another company that appears on *Fortune*'s 100 Best Companies list, reports that almost 90 percent of employees take advantage of flexible work arrangements, including flextime and telecommuting. At Hewlett-Packard Company, the first major corporation to introduce flextime in 1972, employees at all locations have access to flexible work arrangements, and most U.S. workers at HP take advantage of it. Not surprisingly, HP also appears consistently on the *Fortune*'s and *Working Mother*'s 100 Best Companies lists. In hospitals, compressed work weeks have been in effect with mixed results. For a number of years, nurses in many different institutions have worked 12-hour shifts for three days in a given week, essentially working 36 hours while getting paid for 40. The economics of this arrangement have proven challenging from a cost, staffing, and continuity perspective. As a result, hospitals that once embraced the arrangement are going back to more traditional approaches and requiring a full work week.

Telecommuting, where employees essentially work from home, has become another popular option in many non-healthcare companies. At Prudential Insurance Company, although 15,000 employees in 2000 tapped flex programs, 12,000 workers telecommuted from home. McDonald's reports that 37 percent of its management and staff at its Oak Brook, Illinois, headquarters work flexible schedules, some by telecommuting. Unlike some of their peers, employees at McDonald's receive full benefits if they work at least 20 hours per week, and benefits are prorated for fewer hours.

Given that so many employees engage in flextime and telecommuting, how well do these benefits really work? For some telecommuters, productivity actually increases because telecommuting allows concentration on the task at hand without the office distractions of continuously ringing phones or coworkers "popping" in. However, home distractions may be as significant as work distractions. Thus, success requires significant discipline. As a testimony to telecommuting's popularity, the home office, complete with ergonomically correct office furniture, computer, and fax line, has become a staple in many houses. In many cases, employers provide the computer and pay an allowance toward set up and furniture. VISA USA, in addition to providing generous time-off benefits for new parents, offers flexible scheduling options to all employees, with telecommuters receiving free equipment and a $500 furniture allowance. IBM Corporation, another regular on *Working Mother's* list over the last 16 years, reports that 81,000 of its employees telecommute. To achieve this, the company provides an entire office, including all office furniture, fax machines, dedicated phone lines, and ThinkPads, for all who work full time at home.

As attractive as this option may seem, of course, there are limitations in the translation of this policy to healthcare. Clinical, technical, and environmental support staff, to name but a few departments, would be challenged to provide their services remotely!

Two other family-friendly options include job sharing and working part time. With job sharing, two employees typically share the hours and responsibilities for one position. Although overhead coordination time typically adds to the total cost of the job, there are clear advantages to having employees who want less-than-full-time work. Despite the cost, the most progressive companies allow employees to job share and work part time while still maintaining some level of benefits and remaining on a career track for advancement. At American Management Systems, a business and infotech consulting firm in Fairfax, Virginia, more than 90 percent of employees work flexible schedules, 35 percent to 40 percent work from home, and 5 percent job share.

Johnson & Johnson and AstraZeneca both have endorsed job sharing and part-time work. In fact, both are shining examples of family-friendly companies. Johnson & Johnson's (J&J) former CEO, Ralph Larsen, was personally committed to helping employees balance their lives, carrying on a long-standing corporate value. Throughout his 38-year tenure at J&J, he supported many family-friendly programs, including on-site child care centers, lactation rooms, a job-guaranteed year off for new parents, generous adoption benefits ($5,000 per child), flexible work schedules, and employee assistance programs complete with extensive resource and referral services. For its child care centers, J&J paid the start-up costs and contributes up to 43 percent to their operating costs. Participating employees receive discounts based on income and the number of children they have enrolled. Grandchildren are also eligible for enrollment. Those unable to use these centers receive a 10 percent subsidy toward the cost of other child care options. The company has instituted summer camps for children of its employees, a benefit that E.R. Squibb and Sons—now part of Bristol-Myers Squibb—offered in the 1960s. Although J&J has a hard-working culture, its managers have been trained to be flexible about last-minute requests for time off from their employees, and employees are encouraged to ask for breaks when they need them. Other family-friendly benefits at J&J include work at home, a benefit enjoyed by 23,000 employees in 2000. Another 8,500 employees took advantage of compressed work weeks in 2000. As part of its commitment, J&J holds frequent national seminars that showcase how to promote work-life balance and offers managers training on these topics.

SAS Institute, a computer software company based in North Carolina, also provides family-friendly benefits. Employees are encouraged to work 35-hour weeks, 7-hour days. At its headquarters, a fitness center equipped with soccer and softball fields, jogging trails, basketball courts, a swimming pool, and 17 full-time staff provides stress reduction. Several on-site and near-site day care centers provide child care. Breastfeeding mothers wear beepers to alert them when their babies require their attention. Lactation rooms offer lunch service for mothers. Break rooms are stocked with drinks and snacks, and dry-cleaning services and an on-site hair salon are available. Employees in outlying offices receive substantial financial assistance for child care, paying only $250 a month. For all its efforts, SAS Institute experienced an employee turnover rate of only 5 percent in 1999 in an industry that was averaging 20 percent. The company estimates annual savings of $75 million in recruiting and training costs. Not surprisingly, SAS appears in the number three position on the 2002 *Fortune's* 100 Best Companies to Work For list, down from the number two position in 2001. SAS has been recognized by *Working Mother*s as one of the 100 Best Companies for 12 consecutive years.

AstraZeneca prides itself on its commitment to family-friendly benefits. According to Teresa Bien (2002), director of medical affairs-training at AstraZeneca, not only does the company provide subsidies for the costs of child care, summer camp, and holiday care, they also subsidize back-up child care through their Just in Time program. If a nanny or other caregiver isn't able to care for an employee's child, AstraZeneca foots the bill for an alternative care arrangement, and the same holds true for sick child care. AstraZeneca offers other programs aimed at work-life balance issues. Work weeks, for example, have been reduced from 40 to 37 and one-half hours per week. Compressed work weeks can be designed by the employee in conjunction with his or her manager, structuring a customized arrangement to fit the individual's schedule as long as it doesn't interfere with customer requirements. In some cases, employees work extra time on Monday through Thursday and then take every other Friday off. Telecommuting is a practice supported by funds allocated for extra phone lines or

T1/DSL installation. The company's overall benefit package is generous, extended on a prorated basis to those working part time or in a job-sharing situation. Employees receive full benefits at 30 hours per week, a generous threshold for this level of worked hours.

Strategy 10: Providing Succession and Career Pathing

In Chapter 3, we discussed the results of the top-100 hospital retention survey. In that survey "preference to internal promotion" ranked as the most effective retention tool among participants. The power of internal promotion as a retention tool is significant, and its significance has been recognized by other industries. However, merely focusing on preference to internal promotion fails to leverage this strategy's potential. To really support internal promotion, formal mechanisms must be in place to provide aggressive succession and career pathing. Allstate Insurance Company has a unique mentoring program in that managers and directors are matched with senior executives from other corporations. The idea behind this is that a manager is less inhibited about discussing career aspirations with an outsider. Although many companies do an excellent job in this area, J&J has a unique approach that is consistently implemented across all its 197 autonomous operating units. We've chosen to illustrate what can be done through J&J's experience.

At J&J, individual development plans are designed by employees and their managers within their individual operating unit. Each receives the personalized attention one might expect in a small company. Individual planning occurs through formalized discussions focused on development needs. Discussions then focus on assessing individuals' readiness for promotion, centering on what skills need to be developed to enable the individual to move forward. Skill identification is guided by the companywide Standards of Leadership, the common framework that defines competencies all individuals must exhibit across the business to be effective leaders. Creation of individual development plans, called the "*i*-Lead" process, is multistep and multidimensional. In this model, the individual, manager, and organization each has a role in providing input into the plan.

A related process called succession planning has been evolving at J&J for over 30 years. This process involves intense commitment by management throughout the organization, requiring attendance at the annual three- or four-day retreats focused specifically on succession planning. In this model, senior management on down must identify potential leaders and successors. These managers have the opportunity to demonstrate and "market" their candidates' potential through the system. It is, in effect, both bottom up as well as top down. Structured career paths are well documented and include the particular requirements needed for advancement (e.g., sales and marketing executive ladder, scientific career ladder, and quality career ladder). Cross-functional paths are also defined. To advance within the sales management structure, for example, sales, marketing, and product management experience are all critical. The purpose behind this approach is simple and straightforward. Managers must demonstrate breadth in related areas before advancing. Avenues for advancement must also be available for those not interested in management. In either case, J&J's culture requires that managers and incumbents be actively engaged in the process.

One career path that has received considerable attention in healthcare is the clinical ladder for nurses. In most clinical ladders, levels identify and recognize increasing expertise in clinical practice. They also define which specific criteria enable progress to the next level, both in terms of advancement and compensation (Fitzsimons and Numerof 1997). As nurses climb the clinical ladder, hospitals are expected to offer comprehensive development activities to support progression. Despite the relatively pervasive nature of clinical ladders, not all are well supported nor do they all reflect strategic role priorities. Perhaps most importantly, hospitals must ensure that nursing is not the only function being developed. They must also ensure systematic development for their managers. Succession planning and development must be relevant for more groups of employees. Managers should be held accountable for developing successors and promoting qualified, internal candidates.

Strategy 11: Tracking Organizational Exits as a Tool for Rapid Remediation

Tracking terminations by reason of separation is one approach for controlling turnover that was noted by many top-100 hospital survey respondents. Getting a handle on this requires systematic identification of the actual reason for leaving, either through exit interviews or follow-up calls conducted by human resources or an objective third party. The patterns that emerge from these interviews serve as a starting point for understanding the problem and designing solutions. These patterns give hospitals insight into which issues to address and help them assess the relative effectiveness of current retention-related initiatives. There may also be a side benefit to the calls. Some departing employees are actually re-recruited during the process of talking through why they're leaving. When they do stay, they typically opt to work in a different area from the one they left.

If hospitals are committed to understanding turnover, then they need to slice the data into categories. The first category and subsequent analysis should compare the results of controllable to non-controllable exit data. This provides clearer indicators of areas where the organization may affect termination decisions (e.g., working conditions, compensation, benefits, management). The hospital can then establish priorities to address the causes of turnover, based on areas they can control. Once the broad categories or reasons for leaving are understood, it is important to drill down and review terminations by department to establish patterns emerging from particular areas. Once patterns have been identified, solutions can be developed. Examining terminations by department or unit also provides accountability at the appropriate level, allowing for management bonuses to be at-risk based on results. As noted before, first-line management has the most direct impact on an employee's propensity to leave. As such, managers need to be held accountable for employee movement from their areas.

The impact of turnover monitoring at the unit level shouldn't be underestimated, as the following example suggests. The coauthor of this book (Michael Abrams) established a turnover system at Citigroup, an organization that was experiencing high turnover in the early 1980s. The average tenure at the time was only 23 months, a clear indication that there was a problem with retention. As head of program evaluation and metrics for the Western Hemisphere Management Education group at the headquarters of the consumer finance subsidiary, Abrams observed that turnover tracking was an elective process, not mandated by the organization. When it was tracked, it was for the corporation as a whole and not by the vice president or at the functional manager level. Although managers expressed concern regarding high turnover, there was no accountability for it and no targets or consequences were associated with turnover. Starting with the idea "you can't manage what you're not measuring," Abrams developed a system that measured turnover by manager on a monthly basis then calculated it for the year. Abrams disseminated the results to senior management, who were then forced to acknowledge problem areas and address issues. According to Abrams, "because you were shining a light on the phenomenon, those areas that showed more variability received more attention." The final result was a decrease in turnover rates and an increase in length of tenure. Today, Citigroup is among the top ten companies on the *Working Mother*'s list and has appeared on this list for 11 years.

Assuming exit interviews are on the organization's agenda, the challenge is how to structure the interview and the data-reduction process. If voluntary, effective exit interviews are structured to elicit enough information to understand the reasons an employee is leaving and are based on seeking areas to improve the organization. If involuntary, this approach clarifies any misunderstandings to avoid potential legal problems. Although exit interviews can be conducted by human resources or third parties, they should not be conducted by immediate supervisors. Departing employees are reluctant to honestly report their reasons for leaving to someone who could have been a primary cause of their departure. As we have argued throughout this book, the direct manager dramatically influences employees' satisfaction and their propensity to stay with the organization.

Having selected who will conduct the interview, the next question is when to conduct it. Interviews can take place immediately after an employee gives notice to leave or immediately prior to the actual departure date. When using a third party, interviews can be conducted after the employee has terminated employment, although this may result in lower response rates. However, waiting until the employee has actually left the organization will not result in any last-minute "saves" because the employee is already out the door.

Once exit interviews are conducted, data should be aggregated and summarized by department. Then, the data must be communicated back to managers and senior executives to determine trends and next steps. If data trends suggest remedial action, changes should be implemented as soon as possible to stop preventable turnover down the road.

We should point out that some people believe that exit interviews are ineffective and therefore is a waste of scarce resources. Critics point to a number of problems; one argument lands squarely on the interviewer. Essentially, this criticism finds fault with the fact that the interviewer only knows the employee through files and is therefore unlikely to elicit personal information and feelings. Along the same lines, critics argue that employees are circumspect and will not reveal negative information about the company to maintain a congenial relationship that essentially ensures that they don't "burn their bridges." Another argument is that results will not be portrayed accurately to the manager, which results in the wrong actions being taken to correct deficiencies or worse yet, no action at all. Finally, critics maintain that exit interviews don't actually improve the quality of worklife once the decision to leave the organization has been made. Given that problems should have been explored and resolved during employment, critics contend that an exit interview is a little like closing the barn door after all the horses have left.

From our perspective, none of these arguments is a good enough reason not to conduct exit interviews. Let's start with the barn door analogy first. Although it is true that nothing can be done to improve the departing employee's past experience, lessons learned from that experience can systematically be used to improve the work experience of current and future employees. In select cases, appropriate concern and transfer may in fact save an exit. Assuming a good exit interview protocol and good interviewing skills on the part of the interviewer, the fact that the interviewer doesn't know the employee may lead to better probing analysis and insight. Strong interviewing skills will solicit honest feedback without putting the employee at risk, especially when confidentiality is promised; this is an argument for outsourcing the process. Finally, it is management's responsibility to do something with the results, including providing constructive feedback and guidance to managers who are experiencing high turnover. Failure to do so is akin to failing to take action when finances are headed south or quality indicators point to problems.

CONCLUSION

One final note on lessons learned in other industries: Enron, the energy giant, was among *Fortune*'s 100 Best Companies in 2001. At the beginning of 2001, the company reported that it was experiencing 30 percent job growth and had offered extensive training and generous starting salaries for new employees. It gave all employees stock options when the stock price hit $50 a share and was rewarded with a nominal 6 percent voluntary turnover rate, a sure sign of loyal employees. However, Enron has now filed for the largest bankruptcy in U.S. history and the "generous" stock options are now virtually worthless. On the surface, this company may have been a model for best practices, but in reality it obviously is not. Financial and general business integrity must be the umbrella under which all benefits and retention practices are developed.

Assuming such integrity exists, then the lesson to be learned here is that each organization must decide which recruitment and retention practices will work best for it. They must be realistic, focus on short-term and long-term goals, and take into account what is practical for the organization. The dynamics in healthcare, where stock does not exist, obviously preclude stock options from being an available benefit for employees. Telecommuting isn't realistic when staff members need to care for patients in the hospital. However, other practices can be replicated that will increase retention, as long as they fit within the structural, cultural, and financial parameters of the healthcare organization. At a minimum, this chapter certainly helps us to see what's possible.

As we look at cross-industry practices, one significant lesson stands out: Truly, the best-in-class have created a brand, one that endures during hard times and plentiful times. Those organizations that have been cited here as exemplars maintained their commitment to their employees even during very difficult economic times, taking a long-term view of their workforce. In contrast, we described many healthcare organizations that take a short-term view. These institutions recruit and terminate employees based on short-term fluctuations in business. They unwittingly create a short-term mindset in employees that is driven by an hourly mentality.

From creating and leveraging the brand through targeted incentives and recognition and communication programs to ensuring managerial accountability for retention and family-friendly benefits, the 11 winning strategies offer healthcare organizations insight into effective recruitment and retention. Although these are important ingredients for attracting and retaining the workforce, there are additional steps organizations must take to ensure success.

These are described next in Chapter 7. They enable and ensure that a brand of excellence is an operational reality.

REFERENCES

Air Force News. 2000. "Air Force Turns Focus to Recruiting, Retention in 2000." *Air Force News* (January 4).

Anderson, C. 2002. Interview with authors.

Bien, T. 2002. Interview with authors.

Bilbrey, P. 2002. Interview with authors.

Breitenbach, T. 2002. Interview with authors.

Case, E. 2002. Interview with authors.

The Chicago Tribune. 1999. "Employees Becoming Key Recruitment Tools." *The Chicago Tribune* (August 13).

Clapp, J. R., Jr. 2002. Interview with authors.

The Dallas Morning News. 2000. "Employee-Referral Incentive Programs Pay Off for Dallas-Area Hospitals." *The Dallas Morning News* (September 17).

Fitzsimons, S., and R. E. Numerof. 1997. "Educating Nurses for the Future." In *The Executive Nurse,* edited by S. R. Byers. Albany, NY: Delmar Publishers.

Fortune. 2001. "The 100 Best Companies to Work For." *Fortune* (January 22).

———. 2002. "The 100 Best Companies to Work For." *Fortune* (February 4).

Monster.com. 2001. "IT Retention Strategies: Saving HR Time and Money." [Online article; retrieved 12/29/01]. www.monster.com.

Philadelphia Inquirer. 2001. "School Board Votes to Use Bonuses to Fight Teacher Gap." *Philadelphia Inquirer* (March 27).

Regier, A. 2002. Interview with authors.

San Jose Mercury News. 2000. "Employee, Employers Alike Reap Rewards from Referral Programs." *San Jose Mercury News* (July 11).

Smith, B. 2002. Interview with authors.

Trustee. 2000. "Rolling Out the Red Carpet for Employees." *Trustee* (February 15).

Working Mother. 2001. "100 Best Companies for Working Mothers." *Working Mother* (October).

Chapter 7

Successful
Strategy Execution

HEALTHCARE DELIVERY IS at a crossroads. The issues surrounding current staffing needs have reached a critical point and threat-
en to jeopardize the quality and safety of patient care delivery. The
challenge of improving recruitment and increasing retention in
today's turbulent healthcare environment is formidable. This task
increasingly becomes more difficult daily. Effectively reducing
turnover, however, requires more than increasing salaries, offering
bonuses, and conducting meetings. Given the complex nature of
the problem, only integrated, systemic initiatives will succeed.

What is necessary for hospitals to do to reverse the current exodus of talent is a systematic rethinking of assumptions about how
healthcare organizations are designed and structured. What follows is our blueprint for moving your organization forward.

REDEFINING MISSION AND VISION

Although the problems discussed in earlier chapters are common in
all hospitals, the path to change must be developed one hospital at
a time. It begins with a strategic review of the hospital's position in

the marketplace—that is, its competitive stature, historic strengths, the nature of its patient population and their expectations, its financial position, and the identification of what it must deliver to its various constituencies to be successful. Concurrently, an analysis must be completed to arrive at an objective understanding of the underlying issues behind recruiting, retention, quality, and satisfaction problems. Such efforts require, at a minimum, structured interviews with a range of players who can offer insight—that is, current and former staff, administrators, physicians, and patients. Most important though is that this strategic reassessment must take place in a context of genuine openness and with a commitment to "think out of the box." Old agendas and assumptions must be put aside, and it must be made clear to those whose input is solicited that they are being invited to say what they really think, not to repeat the conventional wisdom or the politically acceptable point of view.

What should emerge from this strategic reassessment is a new, clearer vision for patient care. Even when the analysis suggests that the prevailing view is substantially on target, a determined effort to revalidate direction should be a unifying and energizing experience, yielding new clarity on the few things that matter the most.

BLUEPRINT FOR BECOMING AN EMPLOYER OF CHOICE

Strategic reassessment and commitment to a new patient care vision set the stage for rethinking core elements of the way that the organization functions. We have concluded that there are six "pillars" that support patient care effectiveness and that are necessary to attract and retain quality employees.

1. *Ensure role clarity* through job charters and competencies that define expectations of individuals' roles and their role on a multidisciplinary team.
2. *Establish optimal structures, focus on clear accountability for excellence, and provide support for development to achieve goals.*

3. *Establish excellent core processes and standardize practices* that cut across all services to increase efficiency, increase effectiveness, and lower costs, building in custom processes where needed.
4. *Ensure real-time availability of appropriate equipment, supplies, and tools* to deliver excellence.
5. *Create a patient-centered environment* where safety, cleanliness, customer service, and excellence in patient outcomes are expected and delivered reliably.
6. *Design multiple patient care delivery models* that meet the needs of distinctly different patient populations.

These six pillars present problem clusters that we have found repeatedly over 20 years of consulting and employee survey experience to consistently correlate with high levels of turnover and with problematic implementation of effective patient care. In the discussion that follows, we have outlined what each pillar involves, the circumstances that typically create the problem cluster, and the implications for fixing them.

PILLAR 1: ENSURE ROLE CLARITY

The Issue

At its simplest level, much of role clarity is captured by the answer to the survey question "To what extent do you understand what is expected of you in your job?" In many hospitals, employees really are not clear on this. For a variety of reasons, the scope of their jobs seems to vary from day to day, unit to unit, and with the management intervention of the month.

Another major component of role clarity is captured in the question "To what extent do you understand how what you do makes a difference in meeting the objectives of the hospital?" In Chapter 5, we discussed the devolution of roles to the tactical level. The consequence of this devolution is that over time, employees lose sight of the larger goals of the institution and rely on their own preferences and values to guide them under conditions of uncertainty. They do what is most gratifying, most comfortable, and most familiar to them but not necessarily what the hospital needs from them to be successful.

Lack of role clarity constrains organizational effectiveness by dissipating effort in nonconstructive ways. It also sets the stage for higher levels of stress. Clear role definition and identification of the critical interfaces for each role provide the basis for understanding and setting expectations for each individual and their respective positions. Identification of individual responsibility in a collaborative and multidisciplinary team culture must be documented and communicated. Clarity of roles provides the basis for systematic measurement, monitoring, and improvement of performance. At a fundamental level, lack of role clarity introduces ambiguity and stress into the work environment and dramatically increases the likelihood of mismatches between expectation and performance. Job satisfaction, and ultimately employee retention, hangs in the balance along with related effects on unit stability, the cumulative knowledge base, and patient satisfaction.

How We Got Here

A variety of experiments in the restructuring of healthcare staffing intended to lower costs have brought us to this current situation. The most common experiment was to translate reengineering concepts directly from a manufacturing environment to that of healthcare delivery.

Throughout the 1990s, many hospital administrators attempted to take a page from the cost-cutting playbook of manufacturing by parceling out the elements of the registered nurse role that RNs weren't required by law to do to unlicensed healthcare providers. The case for doing so was compelling. Anticipated benefits included:

- the RN could provide a narrower range of higher-level activities to a greater number of patients,
- basic tasks that RNs preferred not to do would be handed off,

- patient care would be coordinated by the RN, who was in the best position to know what was needed and when,
- coordination by the RN would allow their managers to effectively manage larger spans of control,
- reduction in the RN-to-patient ratio would lower overhead costs, and
- a career path would be created for unlicensed healthcare providers.

Unfortunately, poor implementation and a variety of unanticipated consequences have in many cases meant that these benefits did not materialize, and, in fact, staff retention suffered as a result.

One of the biggest negative effects of this strategy was that it put nurses in a pseudo-supervisory role. The assumption that nurses would coordinate the efforts of these unlicensed caregivers around the needs of their patients was rarely examined carefully. In fact, most nurses were not equipped, either by training or by inclination, to take on such a task. Their lack of preparedness to deal with supervisory issues was exacerbated in many situations by cultural differences between the nursing cadre and those they were expected to oversee. The former group was educated and socio-economically mainstream, the latter had limited education and work experience and tended to be minority and poor. For many nurses, the net result was simply "not what they got into nursing to do."

A further complication was that the supply of support caregivers almost never met the projected need. A tight labor market, marginally competitive compensation, and requirements for evening and weekend hours made recruiting and retention a problem. Turnover of between 40 percent and 60 percent was not uncommon. Meanwhile, the nurse-to-patient staffing ratio was adjusted upward to account for the time that had been freed up from the nursing role, generally without regard for the reality that these "extenders" were in many cases nothing more than approved openings. Nurses who were in touch with the needs of their patients generally chose to deliver service themselves rather than force their patients to wait for the "right" caregiver to become available. An 8-hour or 12-hour shift of trying to be a nurse, nurse extender, and pseudo-supervisor has helped many nurses reach the decision to "vote with their feet."

The consequences of force-fitting nurses into a pseudo-supervisory role have been insidious and the impact has been profound on the nursing population. For those who are still part of the system, the result, in many cases, has been confusion. "Should I do only what regulations require? Or should I do what extenders and inadequately staffed support departments leave undone?" In some hospitals, the pressure to do what's needed for adequate patient care makes meaningful role definition impossible. Managers stretched across untenable spans of control don't offer much clarification. For many nurses, this ambiguity threatens their sense of professional identity and makes the hospital environment less and less attractive.

Although the consequences of ill-advised cost-reduction tactics have had their most dramatic impact on nurses, such consequences have not been limited to that group. Among support staff groups, the pressure to reduce costs has translated into fewer staff and often a "what services can the hospital do without" orientation. As a result, staffing levels are often not sufficient to provide services in a timely way. Requests to central supply for equipment and linens go unheeded because no one is available to bring them to the unit. Medical equipment that needs repair or adjustment backs up in repair queues, and functioning equipment on the floor becomes increasingly scarce. Working supervisors are forced to be "another pair of hands" to cope with the workload, and such activities as process improvement and employee coaching and development go by the board.

Action Items

The challenge in addressing role clarity is to build consensus among role incumbents and their managers on an understanding of the job that is consistent across the hospital and that delivers what the hospital needs to achieve its strategic objectives. This new understanding of the role must clarify those elements that have been muddied over the years such as the strategic relevance of the position or "purpose," key accountabilities, decision-making authority, and primary interfaces.

The key to developing this new consensus lies in the process used to redefine a role. Such a process must be one that takes a strategic perspective and that involves role incumbents and their managers in the activity. We have developed a process for this purpose that we call job chartering. Job chartering is the suggested intervention of choice for ensuring job clarity, whether the job is that of an individual contributor or a manager, from nursing through all the support areas of the hospital. Here are some of the key elements of the process.

Start by selecting a design team of 8 to 12 people who represent experienced, strong performers in the role and managers in the role. Members of the design team individually complete a short written questionnaire first, allowing each member to reflect on the position and its responsibilities. Subsequently, the design team comes together and, with the help of a facilitator, works toward consensus on the questionnaire and each section of the job charter. Job charters include sections that detail the strategic relevance of each role, key accountabilities, key interfaces, and the level of decision-making authority for each position. The facilitator takes copious notes and then creates the draft charter for review by the design group. Following review and consensus, incumbent meetings are held to review the document and provide cross-functional perspective on the role. Proposed modifications and their implications are then discussed and debated by the design group. Approved changes are incorporated into the draft document. Finally, the job charter is completed and communication of the finished document is planned and implemented. Although this document is the primary, tangible output of the job charter process, the interaction between and buy-in of incumbents and their managers is the most critical outcome for successful implementation.

To create buy-in and build a case for change based on data, we recommend conducting an activity study. The purpose of an activity study is to capture and summarize how incumbents currently spend their time on the job. This is done by having a sample of incumbents, who are typically recognized as high performers, keep a time log in which they record their activities. The data are summarized by category and then discussed with the sample in the context of the newly designed job charter. One advantage of this process is that it forces an examination of what people *are* doing and not what they *think* they are doing, framing the problem-solving process around data analysis rather than competing opinions. The activity study enables incumbents to focus on the way time is currently spent and compare it to the way time will be spent if the new job charter were in place. Activity study shines a spotlight on the gap between the current and future state and sets the stage for meaningful planning to close that gap.

The tangible outputs of the job-charter process are documents that specify the boundaries and expectations of roles. It's natural for practitioners to want to leverage the work of others and perhaps use a charter developed elsewhere; this is a mistake for at least two reasons. First of all, it is dangerous to assume that one size fits all. Each hospital has its own history, culture, and mission and each needs to craft roles that take those factors into consideration. The most important outcome of the job-charter process is the engagement of incumbents and their managers in a process that requires them to look at the role in a strategic context. The consensus that results from such a process is the binding force that sets the stage for meaningful follow-through. No job charter borrowed from another organization can make this happen.

Creating a job charter for a particular role should not be the end of the process. Once a job charter has been created and agreed on, competencies for ensuring successful performance should be articulated. Competencies describe the behaviors that job incumbents must be capable of delivering to achieve overall success in the position. Each key accountability in the job charter is associated with specific competencies that make achievement of that accountability possible. For example, to successfully deliver on the key accountability of providing consistent vision and leadership to staff, job incumbents logically need to be able to articulate policy guidelines to staff using terms and a communication style that ensures understanding and encourages buy-in.

Once competencies have been drafted, reviewed, and agreed on by incumbents and their managers, they should be incorporated into an integrated performance management process and professional development program. Because they are framed in behavioral terms, competencies translate easily into these processes, ensuring consistency and strategic focus. Beyond this, using competencies in this way provides managers with the tools to have more meaningful dialog with employees about expectations, performance feedback, and development opportunities. A clear understanding of the competencies involved in a particular job provides critical input for both the selection process and organizationwide succession planning.

Alignment of the performance management, development, and selection processes is an important longer-term outcome of the process. We have also seen dramatic changes in effectiveness resulting from more clearly defined roles and strategic focus. This has led to higher levels of job satisfaction and increased retention levels.

The question of where in the organization we can start to apply an approach like job chartering is a fairly easy one. As we discussed in Chapter 5, the role of the patient care manager is at the center of the action. The core infrastructure of the role must be addressed, focusing on educational needs, advanced clinical practice support, managerial and administrative support, etc. Clarifying the purpose and identifying expectations and accountabilities of all members of the delivery team to each other and the patients are the first steps in improving retention of experienced employees.

Although the case can be made that nursing has the greatest vulnerability and so must be given the highest priority for role clarification, it is important to understand that because clinical care delivery is such a specialized and interdependent process, support functions must also be addressed to make the changes for nursing viable. Development of job charters for these critical jobs is an effective vehicle for establishing this clarity. For the managers, clear accountability for retention must be among their charters' key accountabilities to properly position them in the context of improving retention.

Over the past 20 years of our consulting work, we have found that a job-charter development process is the most powerful way of addressing the role ambiguity that afflicts many healthcare organizations today. Effectively extending the process by developing competencies and weaving them into employee development, performance appraisal, selection, and succession planning will help hospitals catch up their human resources processes with the best practices of world-class organizations outside the healthcare business. In our client organizations, we have seen dramatic changes in effectiveness, even early in the process. The fact that systemic action is being taken to provide structure around such fundamental sources of discomfort is in itself a significant boost to morale. Ultimately, the consistent articulation and alignment of role requirements with organizational objectives increases predictability in an environment that desperately needs more.

PILLAR 2: ESTABLISH OPTIMAL STRUCTURE AND ACCOUNTABILITY

The Issue

The issue of structure in healthcare today is, at its most basic level, based on numbers. In hospital after hospital across the country, the span of control in nursing has been increased to the point that it's not uncommon to find nurse managers responsible for supervising between 100 and 200 nurses. The principal driver of this trend is the need to cut cost, and supervisory salaries are a visible and convenient target. Such tactics have been justified in part by the decentralization of supervisory responsibilities to nurses themselves. After all, if nurses are "coordinating" the efforts of their extenders and fewer nurses are available, then fewer supervisors are needed to oversee the situation. Another argument that has been used to rationalize the situation is that because nurses are highly trained professionals and put their licenses at risk to fulfill their responsibilities, they need comparatively little oversight.

The assumption that underlies this trend is that availability of a manager to her staff does not make a meaningful difference to the effective operation of the unit on a day-to-day basis. Activity studies conducted in client hospitals suggest that managers' time is increasingly accounted for by administrative duties—that is, managing budget, juggling schedules and time off for staff, negotiating with staff to obtain coverage, and representing the interests of their units in multiple meetings where the criterion for a "good decision" is comprehensive input.

Seen in context of the legacy of "self governance," the reduction of the role of the nurse manager to that of external representative and internal paper shuffler is a logical extension of cultural trends. This contraction of the expected role of managers extends beyond nursing to all facets of the hospital. Unfortunately, it represents change in a direction that offers employees less support at a time when what they need is more.

The issue of accountability is not quite so easily observable, but it is equally problematic as an obstacle to employee retention. The simple fact is that at a time when patients are becoming more and more sensitive to the quality of their hospital experience, the quality of performance by nurses and non-nursing staff alike seems to matter less and less. There are several reasons for this.

One reason that performance seems increasingly unconnected to consequences is there is more limited supervision. After performing administrative and representational duties, the average manager has little time left. With spans of control adding up to three digits, the nursing manager will not likely get to see a meaningful sample of any employee's performance, either positive or negative. This typically doesn't stop managers from conducting performance appraisals, but it does raise credibility issues regarding whatever judgments are made in that appraisal process.

Another reason is related to the shortage of personnel in the industry. In many cases, managers would rather have a mediocre performer—anybody—than nobody at all. Glossing over performance shortfalls has become an increasingly common practice in many hospitals, as the short-term cost of taking corrective action appears to outweigh the short-term cost of inaction. The long-term cost that is frequently overlooked is the corrosive impact on administration's credibility on the subject of standards and service and on the motivation of stronger performers who logically ask themselves "why bother?"

A third reason is that in most hospital environments, there is little real-time feedback of a positive nature and performance appraisal systems are typically insensitive to meaningful performance differences. Because managers have so little opportunity to actually observe first hand the performance of their employees, feedback tends to be based on negative exceptions. When something goes wrong or someone complains, a report is made, an investigation is conducted, and sanctions sometimes are administered. This provides little opportunity for positive feedback, and none of it happens in real time. Performance appraisals conducted by managers who are far removed from actual performance observation typically incorporate so many other factors, such as completion of educational requirements and even community service, that the few critical things that matter in the realm of quality and service get lost in the mix.

Finally, current compensation systems, designed more to mollify the workforce than to differentiate between performance levels, make such minimal distinctions between mediocre and high performers that any incentive for aspiring to excellence must come from elsewhere.

Action Items

All of the issues raised here—demotivation of staff, inconsistent or low standards of performance, and failure of management to address performance gaps—are tied to the curiously contracting role of the healthcare manager. The notion that performance can be continuously improved; that the psychological needs of employees for direction, reinforcement, feedback, etc. can be met; and that staff can be kept informed, motivated, and focused on strategic objectives of the organization without a meaningful managerial presence runs counter to decades of research and experience. Part of the answer here is, once again, in the numbers. How many staff can a manager realistically supervise?

As with most real-world problems, there is no single answer to the span-of-control question. However, guidelines do exist. Figure 7.1 identifies 11 characteristics of the work environment that should be evaluated to arrive at an optimal span of control.

What should be clear from consideration of these characteristics is that appropriate span of control cannot be achieved without some in-depth understanding of the work, the staff, and the manager involved. Virtually no other industry, particularly one in which the work is as variable and unpredictable as in healthcare, attempts to direct employee efforts through spans of control as great as we find in nursing today. As a rule, a broad span of control (for a shift manager, for example) should generally not exceed 20 to 25 employees. This would be subject to expansion or contraction based on the considerations outlined in the figure.

Increasing the availability of managers is part of the solution. At least as important is broadening the understanding of the role that managers can and must play in building a healthcare culture that works. This calls for a radical redefinition of the manager's role, first in the minds of administrators and then through the eyes of managers themselves, using a process like job chartering.

A process that builds a common understanding among managers of their strategic roles, key accountabilities, critical interfaces,

Figure 7.1: Guidelines for Creating Optimal Span of Control

Characteristics	Implications
1. Similarity of the work performed across direct reports	1. Enables broader span of control
2. Complexity of the work (including high acuity, criticality, and patient turnover) produced from the department	2. Requires narrower span of control
3. Relative autonomy/experience of direct reports	3. Enables broader span of control
4. Organizational maturity of direct reports and identification with strategic goals	4. Enables broader span of control
5. Professional maturity of direct reports	5. Enables broader span of control
6. Experience of the manager	6. Enables broader span of control
7. Heterogeneity of the work group	7. Requires narrower span of control
8. Stability of the work process	8. Enables broader span of control
9. Level of development of unit infrastructure (i.e., processes, procedures, role clarity, etc.)	9. Enables broader span of control
10. Extent to which pre-job education versus on-the-job training prepared direct reports to perform the work	10. Enables broader span of control
11. Stability of the work group	11. Enables broader span of control

and decision-making authority will go a long way toward setting the stage for improved retention of staff and increased effectiveness of the delivery process. Beyond establishing a common understanding of what needs to be done, healthcare organizations need to take the necessary steps to build the skills of these managers so that they can, in fact, accomplish those key accountabilities. In healthcare as in most industries there is a tendency to promote people who demonstrate superior technical skills. The result of this practice in nursing, pharmacy, and other clinical areas is that those who become managers command the respect of their people for their technical prowess; but they don't necessarily have the conflict management abilities, influence, coaching, and other skills necessary to be successful as managers. Businesses in other industries spend 2 percent to 4 percent of their gross revenues on employee development, an amount that dwarfs the typical allocation in most healthcare organizations. Attempting to create an environment that attracts and retains talented people with an inadequately resourced management infrastructure is a futile endeavor; trying to do so with an inadequately trained one is only slightly better.

Getting managers and their employees to be on the same page regarding what needs to be done is an important step toward building a more hospitable work environment. Developing consensus on key accountabilities and competencies provides the basis for holding people accountable and systematically developing their capabilities. Giving managers the necessary training to ensure that they are able to coach, counsel, influence, and take action to correct inadequate performance ensures that the right steps can be taken. Building the expectation into managers' roles that action will be taken and giving managers the time and resources to make the action realistic and doable will ensure that change does in fact happen.

PILLAR 3: ESTABLISH CORE PROCESS EXCELLENCE AND STANDARDIZE PRACTICES

The Issue

In spite of the many years they have talked about process reengineering, most healthcare organizations have only begun to scratch the surface when it comes to the core clinical processes that most directly affect their costs and the experience of both their patients and staff. In as much the same way that roles like that of a nurse have come to be defined differently from unit to unit, fundamental processes like documentation management, medication, incident tracking, housekeeping, infection control, admissions and discharge and others have been "locally grown," or individually "reinvented" but never really rationalized, standardized, and managed for process improvement across the organization. The common response to this idea is "Sure that's a good idea, but we're different!" Although it's true that the business of healthcare delivery is too complex to be treated as a monolithic activity, this fact doesn't rule out a common core to each process with concessions to unique local conditions "bolted on."

The consequence of the process proliferation that has historically flourished in most hospital organizations is that it raises the psychological and real costs for any person (or process) who crosses over unit boundaries. The float pool, transfers, travelers, and those who are just filling in must all deal with the extra stress of learning "how we do things here." Patients moved from one area to another must adjust to different ways of getting what they need. The variability itself contributes cost, rework, opportunities for errors and misunderstandings, and stress to an environment that is intrinsically unpredictable. This level of process variability contributes to our current retention problems.

The other consequence of this situation is that process improvement—the systematic study of process effectiveness—becomes increasingly expensive and burdensome as the range of applicability grows smaller. The prospect of cutting 5 percent off the cycle time for all pain medication deliveries across the hospital makes intensive study of the process worthwhile. If each unit has a unique delivery process, however, operating costs rise and the payoff shrinks accordingly. Suddenly it seems like not such a great idea; besides, everyone on the unit is so busy anyway.

Action Items

Management and staff must work together, for the good of the institution, to review practices that increase efficiency and effectiveness and lower costs through the use of best practices and innovation. Custom or unique processes can be addressed where needed once core processes are optimized and standardized. Identification of the common or joint processes that most directly affect clinical outcomes and that are at the heart of hospital operations is necessary for the continued success of the institution.

Ideally a group of cross-functional, mid-level or high-level managers led by a facilitator will identify and prioritize the processes to be reviewed. Our bias is to begin with a limited number of processes that create high vulnerability for the organization from the perspective of cost, quality, employee, or customer satisfaction. Next, the group will assemble appropriate documentation to make the case for action, present a proposal for review that outlines which processes will be addressed and what potential impact they will present to the organization, and gain approval from top management. This set of steps, often overlooked in a redesign project, enhances the opportunity for success. Up-front agreement on which processes to review eliminates one obstacle to final approval.

After decisions have been made on what processes will be reviewed and senior management is in agreement on the importance of each selected process, individuals from various backgrounds and organizational levels should be identified to work as a group in reviewing each process. Process maps are systematically defined, illustrating the gaps and inefficiencies in the current process. Assumptions are challenged; for example, does the cardiologist need to review each ER patient before admission when 99 percent of the time the ER physician's guidance is medically correct? What would happen if patients were admitted directly for treatment? Baseline costs, quality, and cycle-time effects are determined, providing data for resource reallocation that are in the best long-term interests of the organization. What is being done today that is no longer applicable? What can be standardized? How can necessary work be made more efficient? Which processes are unique and need to be addressed as singular entities? Each review group has a responsibility to ask these questions as well as other appropriate questions.

Based on the factual information collected and review of the activities within the process, recommendations for change are made.

These recommendations are reviewed by a team composed of those affected by the changes. Proposed modifications and the resulting effects are considered by the review team and incorporated where possible. The result is a set of recommendations that is more likely to be accepted; smoothly implemented; and has significant cost, quality, and cycle-time effects. Management then reviews the final recommendation and implementation plan. Although questions and debate may arise during this process, recommendations following this structured approach are typically approved. Finally, implementation can begin.

Selection of these processes will necessarily vary from institution to institution depending on their focus and where they are most at risk. Clinical pathways, admission and discharge, and development of multidisciplinary plans of care are examples of such focus. Key to success is the prioritization of core process "contenders," a disciplined approach to process redesign, communication, and systematic implementation. Implementation of systematic process management and improvement methodologies made possible by undertaking this task will put hospitals on the path to leveraging the methodologies that other industries have been benefiting from for many years. As important is that it will contribute to making the work environment a more predictable place and, in that regard, will improve the experience of patients and staff.

PILLAR 4: ENSURE REAL-TIME AVAILABILITY OF APPROPRIATE EQUIPMENT, SUPPLIES, AND TOOLS

The Issue

It's ironic that in today's high-tech world of healthcare delivery, where every day we are brought closer to doing what was considered impossible only the day before, caregivers are hamstrung by basic shortages in supplies and equipment. Over the past decade, driven by the same cost pressures noted earlier, hospitals have cut back on staffing support functions. In many organizations, processes for maintenance of equipment and replenishment of supplies on the unit cannot be counted on to ensure the availability of equipment or supplies when needed.

But the problem goes beyond the fact that there aren't enough staff members to fulfill these basic tasks. The deeper problem is that in many institutions managers and employees in support departments have lost sight of the fact that their primary job responsibility is to ensure the smooth flow of services at the patient-interface level. This problem becomes abundantly clear when callers to central supply are told simply that if they want a certain equipment or supply now, they'll need to get it themselves. With the patient and/or doctor watching the clock, it's typically the caregiver—the nurse—who is forced to fill the gap between what's needed and what's available. One consequence of this situation is the proliferation of "private supply stashes"—supplemental emergency inventories of critical items such as catheters, IV needles—to cushion situations when the formal supply has been depleted. As stashing supplies becomes standard practice, inventory costs rise and the term "materials management" becomes an oxymoron.

Beyond cost issues, the greater damage that results is on the psychology of the work environment. Caregivers increasingly feel that they are out there on their own and that the support network that was supposed to be there for them isn't. This failure of the system to live up to its promises erodes employee confidence in the credibility of the system itself, encouraging a cynical, self-protective point of view that undermines employee identification with the organization and confidence in other staff.

Action Items

An initial step in addressing this problem is for senior management to recognize the reality that other industries have been acknowledging for some time: the cost of achieving quality is cheaper than the alternative. The cost—in terms of nursing productivity, patient and physician satisfaction, and turnover—of having nurses chase down critical supplies and equipment is far greater than the cost of having support staff do their jobs. With this perspective as a starting point, an approach such as job chartering in each support area should be undertaken to build a new commitment from managers and support staff to ensure accountability for seamless care delivery at the patient interface.

Concurrent with this role redefinition for support managers and staff, processes for resupply and maintenance of critical materials and equipment should be standardized, streamlined, and calibrated for the specific needs of internal customers. When unit needs, rather than support staffing patterns, drive process configuration, that is an indication that the right steps have been taken. Finally, real-time metrics must be created and monitored that will provide insight into the fulfillment of these new commitments. Such metrics must be linked to timely, appropriate, and meaningful consequences.

The current crisis in healthcare delivery is born out of a labor shortage and economic constraints. To accomplish the necessary changes, institutions must use all resources effectively and support departments need to adequately understand their roles and the environment in which care is currently delivered. No longer can institutions afford to treat areas differently, including or excluding them because of perceived criticality. The success of each healthcare organization depends on recognizing that each unit and each individual make unique contributions and each must be supported and held accountable for making its respective contributions successful.

Staff must be provided with the correct tools; sufficient supplies; and up-to-date, well-maintained equipment to provide excellent patient care. This is not only critical to the health and safety of the patient, it also provides an environment where employees can be proud of the work they do and know that their efforts are supported in the most fundamental ways. Management review of the supply and equipment structure is critical to building and maintaining an environment that employees can be confident will support and complement their work.

PILLAR 5: CREATE A PATIENT-CENTERED ENVIRONMENT

The Issue

All healthcare organizations create an environment for patient care. The quality of that patient environment is critical to clinical outcomes and satisfaction. Clearly, it is incumbent on all organizations to create a patient environment where safety, cleanliness, customer service, and excellence in patient outcomes are expected. Environmental or service associates must understand their criticality and contribution to cleanliness, and health unit coordinators must see why creating a patient-friendly environment helps everyone. Each staff member must be expected to understand his or her role and its relationship to other roles, contribution, and responsibility.

Unfortunately, the same cost-constrained mindset that drove the staff reductions in support departments resulted in cuts of environmental services staff. To a large extent, these staff reductions reflect the same lack of insight into the relationship between the activity involved and the potential impact on patient, physician, and staff satisfaction. The consequence of these staff reductions is a "creeping" redefinition of what actually constitutes "clean." For the same reasons that performance expectations have slipped for nurses, many healthcare organizations have slowly but inexorably become inured to second-class standards in terms of both aesthetics and infection control. There is no better example of this than the hospital executive who, upon learning that a relative was scheduled for admission to her hospital, called environmental services to request a "VIP clean" room. The existence of this double standard—one for "patients" and one for "patients who really matter"—is an acknowledgment of the concessions that many hospital management teams have made, by design or by default, to financial expediency.

One problem these concessions cause is that employees are forced to reconcile the *talk* about the importance of patient satisfaction with the *reality* that they see on a day-to-day basis. The result is that all staff members at some level grow skeptical about the commitment and sincerity behind what management says to them and to their patients. When employees point out the discrepancy and the situation is rationalized by management as a cost-constraint effect, the outcome is corrosive cynicism that taints the employee-hospital relationship in all aspects.

Action Items

Recommendations for changing the current situation involve three elements: (1) role redefinition, (2) standards re-leveling, and (3) monitoring of feedback and performance management.

The role redefinition for environmental services and related staff has as much to do with redefining the role in the minds of other hospital staff. Environmental services positions are an entry point for people with minimal education into a system in which professional credentials are the backbone of the hierarchical structure. Because of this, and because they are often minorities, employees in this function often feel disenfranchised. Just as frequently, hospital management regards this group as peripheral and doesn't bother to try and excite this group or recognize its value.

All of this is completely at odds with the real impact that this employee group can have on patient, employee, and physician responses to the hospital environment. Organizations that have dedicated themselves to being customer centered, like Disney and Ritz Carlton, long ago elevated the importance of those who control environmental factors commensurate with their customer impact. In healthcare, ample evidence indicates that patients, in the absence of sufficient medical knowledge to evaluate the quality of the medical care they receive, judge the quality of their hospital experience by the aspects that they do understand—that is, the hospitality aspects like the cleanliness and condition of the room and the public areas.

What's needed as a foundation for making environmental services more consistently effective is a sincere effort to elevate the importance of this employee segment. Their role in infection control and in the overall satisfaction of patients is more than sufficient reason to make this group feel like a valued part of the healthcare delivery team. We recommend a marketing approach to raise the profile of this group's function. Develop a value proposition for the function that frames its criticality in terms of its impact on patient, physician, and employee satisfaction. Make the case that excellence in patient care starts with environmental services, then promote the message to key internal constituents. These constituents can be involved in task groups that develop universal standards and model rooms and devise processes for evaluating and reporting on effectiveness as discussed below. Environmental services staff members need to be part of local unit meetings, take ownership for their piece of the picture, and work with other members of the team to ensure that the environment they control meets the highest possible standards.

Even as ties to internal constituents are strengthened through a direct-reporting relationship and attendance at unit meetings, attention must be given to upgrading training and technology available to this function. Orientation and training should be centralized to ensure a common core of methods and procedures. Advances in technology also can make the difference between mediocre and excellent performance. Centralized functional environmental services management should be matrixed to retain a regular relationship with staff and provide continued technical support, problem solving, and development.

Concurrent with the external redefinition of the role of the environmental services function, a process such as job chartering should be used with incumbents to rearticulate their role and responsibilities. The end result of such a process is that each staff member will understand his or her role, contribution, responsibility, and relationship to other roles.

The challenge of re-leveling has to do with standardizing and, most important, concretely illustrating what an acceptable clean room or public area looks like. For this purpose we have found that establishing a model patient room is an effective intervention. Basically, this intervention involves setting aside a patient room that has been cleaned and maintained according to standards that have been agreed on by appropriate internal constituents. The model room or model public area becomes a device that is used to educate environmental services staff and others about the environmental standards expected in the hospital. All incumbents in positions that require core patient contact should be oriented to the model room, from how a patient room should look and feel to what should be included in each room to where accessories should be located. This process ensures that expectations are clear, and it prompts what-if discussions that become "teachable moments."

The job chartering process should incorporate input from managers, incumbents, and key constituents. Based on this consensus, checklists that operationalize the criteria for a clean room should be developed for use in monitoring actual performance of environmental services staff. Unit managers should use these checklists to evaluate patient rooms on their unit, and the data from the checklists can be used as a basis for feedback to environmental services staff. Reporting formats need to be simple, quick, and consistent in terms of what is assessed, who performs the assessment, when and how often the assessment is performed, and what the assessment outcome is. Detailed data can show what elements of the cleaning process are working or not working, for all staff and for individuals. This level of feedback can be used to direct individual staff to training or special problem-solving support, and it can signal when current methods and technology need review.

Along with individual feedback on performance, the whole process of environmental management should be the subject of higher-level attention. One recommended vehicle for this is "environmental rounds." Periodic participation of directors and senior management in such reviews gives credibility to the idea that the hospital takes environmental quality seriously.

Finally, feedback and recognition of excellence are as important to improvement as identification of issues. Recognition in the form of a compliment, letter of appreciation, or something material can be used. The form of recognition or reward should be well thought-out and appropriate for the accomplishment. Designing and implementing a process that ensures quick identification and problem resolution yields the best outcomes. Celebrating even small triumphs ensures momentum!

PILLAR 6: DESIGN MULTIPLE PATIENT CARE DELIVERY MODELS

The Issue

Most healthcare organizations today structure patient care delivery around a single, traditional model. That model assumes primary staffing is done by nurses throughout the institution, regardless of the nature of the patient population. In this model, nurses under the direction of a physician provide the thread of continuity in care and all other staff members—respiratory therapists, physical therapists, etc.—serve in the role of transactional consultants. Although patient-to-nurse ratios do vary across care programs/units based on the clinical needs of the patient population (e.g., ICU versus med-surg unit), the unit manager on most units is almost always a nurse. We believe that it's time to reconsider the near monopoly of nursing on these unit-manager roles and evaluate whether alternatives might serve hospitals and patients more effectively.

In the current situation, career paths for non-nursing clinical staff are extremely limited; their opportunities for exposure to management responsibility are few. As important is that unit management perspectives are dominated by nursing, excluding other points of view. This situation tends to reinforce a rigid status hierarchy in most organizations that severely constrains the ambitions of staff without a nursing background and that does not offer these staff members the opportunity to provide genuine continuity of care.

Action Items

Given that the supply of nurses is currently less than the demand and that this situation is likely to get worse before it improves, any approach that can help the available pool of nursing talent become more efficient and effective deserves consideration. One approach that can make a difference involves challenging the current nursing-dominated model of care by introducing non-nursing clinical caregivers into the pool of candidates for the primary clinician and unit management roles. Imagine the ramifications on staffing (and perceived status) when rehab's primary clinician comes out of a rehab discipline or when the primary clinician for vent patients is a respiratory therapist, and so on. In this new model, nurses are part of the integrated care delivery team, but they play a consultative as opposed to a primary role.

The value of this arrangement includes higher levels of professional engagement and thus improved patient outcomes. Implementation begins with identifying patient groups that would gain value from this approach. These groups may include patient populations that are at risk for not having enough clinical coverage—that is, the number of nurses with specialized knowledge is insufficient to provide care safely. In this case, the model may offer a rationale for redeployment of staff from certain areas to others. The model implies that, depending on skill salience, different kinds of professionals can play the lead role in patient care. This approach changes the care model from the current delivery method. At present, individual disciplines provide patient care and frequently with little true collaboration with other professionals. Under a multidisciplinary, patient-population-sensitive model, there will be dialog and planning around staffing options that make sense for the specific group of patients.

Another innovation that we have helped client hospitals introduce involves making the patient and family members a more integral part of the patient's care. As technology makes monitoring, drug administration, and education increasingly common outside of the hospital setting, the role of the primary caregiver in the hospital must change to incorporate these new options. The assumption that the primary caregiver must do it all needs to give way, both to costs and the supply of staff and to the reality that waiting for discharge to make a clean handoff of responsibility is probably not the best course of action for the patient. For example, what happens when patients and families are more directly engaged in planning for and implementing care delivery? What happens when patients take their own blood pressure and monitor other vital signs? The model has already been established in the care of diabetes; it's time to extend it more broadly.

Such innovative, multidisciplinary approaches will work, and it is critical to the continued success of existing institutions that their use be expanded. Effective implementation will not be an easy task. However, rewards to the hospital include improved employee satisfaction and increased retention of critical staff, improved patient outcomes and satisfaction, a potential reduction in labor costs, and improved staffing flexibility as a result of better deployment of staff across disciplines. Any implementation plan must take into account the magnitude and complexity of the challenges associated with this type of major change.

IMPLEMENTING THE BLUEPRINT

With our blueprint and integration model behind us, it's time to get started. Let's begin by describing a composite consulting engagement in a complex healthcare setting that illustrates the problems we've discussed throughout this book, the approach that we are recommending, and the kinds of issues and challenges that are typical under such circumstances.

A Typical Problem Scenario

Metropolitan Healthcare is a major teaching institution in an urban area. With nearly 1,000 beds, Metropolitan is both a significant employer and a dominant player in the healthcare community. Like other institutions in the industry, Metropolitan had been struggling with the problem of recruitment and retention for some time. Nurse recruiting staff were forever behind the curve, "beating the bushes" endlessly for new staff and only vaguely aware that many new hires left in shockingly short order. Senior administrators were frustrated and concerned that the bonuses, salary market adjustments, flexible hours, and improved benefits they had implemented seemed not to be making a dent in the retention problem. In response, they had formed a recruitment and retention committee made up of people who shared their level of concern, such as senior administrators and directors of patient services and directors of human resources, training, and quality.

The committee had scored some significant "wins" by building linkages with regional schools of nursing and introducing some innovative recruitment approaches. But the committee knew that getting people into the institution was only part of the problem. There had been discussions—endless ones, in fact—at the manager level about the reasons that employees left. The spotty exit interviews that managers completed offered an inconclusive picture. Alternative work environments—doctors' offices, surgi-centers, insurance companies, and so on—seemed to be accounting for many of the defections. Some reports were dramatically negative, citing poor working conditions, broken equipment, and unreasonable work demands. However, the team could not reach a consensus on how seriously to take these reports. The one thing they knew for sure was that Metropolitan could not afford the revolving-door situation. They had come to the conclusion that something needed to be done to address the situation.

Going Beyond Band-Aids

The first step in any problem-solving undertaking is to objectively analyze the situation. A common mistake that many management teams make in trying to deal with retention issues is assuming that there is a simple, tactical fix that will have the desired effect. Often based on opinions presented as data or the conventional wisdom of what others have done, such problem-solving efforts often lead to a succession of Band-Aids that drain resources and don't address the systemic roots of the problem.

A meaningful situation analysis entails:

- assessment of the current environment to identify what is and isn't working,
- articulation of what the desired "to-be" scenario looks like,
- specification of the assumptions that underlie the status quo,
- recognition that from such analysis and engaged discussion significant change is needed and will be implemented,
- identification and prioritization of specific changes needed, and
- (ultimately) development of an implementation plan to close the gap.

At the first consultant-facilitated meeting of the recruitment and retention committee of Metropolitan Healthcare, the initial challenge was redefining the scope of the problem. Members needed to give up the idea that some new wrinkle in pay, benefits, or hours would turn the tide. Having made the focus of the problem a strategic one, it soon became clear to the team that it needed to take a fresh look at the context of the problem before attempting to devise solutions.

Through a structured strategic-visioning process, the committee reviewed the hospital mission; comprehensively analyzed the market, their customer base, and the internal and external trends; and identified issues and barriers. To provide a more objective base for decision making, data were systematically gathered through interviews and focus groups, painting a multidimensional picture of conditions for nurses in the institution. Based on a new understanding of what needed to change, the committee created a new vision statement for patient services that represented the group's consensus:

> Deliver patient care excellence in a safe, collaborative, multidisciplinary environment where employees take ownership for maintaining constructive relationships and are valued for their individual contributions.

The decision to define employee retention as a strategic, rather than tactical, issue is critical. In healthcare, as in most industries, there is significant pressure on leaders to take action, preferably by doing something that will immediately fix the problem. The task group charged with addressing this problem needs to have the management support and self-confidence to resist this pressure. If care is taken to communicate to the rest of the organization that the issue has been defined as strategic and that careful thought is being given to it, often the anticipated impatience never materializes.

Change Management Considerations

The committee's articulation of this new vision statement was a preliminary milestone of its effort. The next task for the group was to market test the new vision. Having come to the first planning meeting with the hope of finding a silver bullet and leaving without one, many committee members were afraid that staff would bitterly complain about the systemic solution—that it wouldn't be fast enough or different enough. Over the next 30 days, the committee held briefings with staff to explain its thinking. These briefings were carefully planned, with members equipped with talking points and timing of the rollout to formal and informal sources of influence, to ensure that the committee had a common voice and to address concerns and sources of resistance. Management, physicians, and staff—and their respective concerns—were separately addressed to ensure buy-in. The committee members were pleasantly surprised. Informal enthusiasm for the back-to-basics approach was clear. The staff was relieved at the focus, felt heard, and was eager to see the next steps.

Several factors contribute to early acceptance of the committee's work in our example. First, data were incorporated into the decision-making process. Second, the group's composition was strong. Involvement of key decision makers was a statement that the institution's administration took the problem seriously and was prepared to take meaningful action. Third, the committee was sensitive to the use of influence and the importance of effective communication in the rollout of the new vision statement. Finally, a sense of urgency was established to ensure sustained momentum throughout implementation.

Having successfully developed a base of support for the redefined patient services vision, the committee then developed action plans for closing the gap between the current situation and the situation defined by the new vision. Their research into the problem led the committee members to start by addressing role clarity for patient care managers.

Role Clarification is Job #1

Over the course of two one-day meetings, the design group, made up of eight of the most articulate high performers, discussed and debated what the strategic contribution, key accountabilities, primary interfaces, and decision-making authority of the patient care manager should be. Concurrently, a total of ten patient care managers participated in an activity study to provide data on how they spent their time.

By the third design group meeting, the team had reached consensus on a job charter for the position. The group used that meeting to review the results of the activity study. What the histograms and pie charts showed was dramatically different from the role the group had agreed patient care managers needed to play. The group members were shocked to see that nearly 20 percent of managers' time was being spent on administrative tasks such as typing, filing, and retrieving forms and reports. The managers spent no time on coaching their staff and almost no time on being coached by their directors or working and managing relationships with physicians on their units. This was how the most effective patient care managers functioned!

One of the real values of an activity study is that it highlights the gaps between what is and what needs to be. Typically, this study prompts meaningful discussion about how such gaps can be closed. Even if the resources are not available immediately, it is critical that the project team develop a plan that over time will address the issue, get the plan approved, or work with administration until some reasonable compromise is reached.

Making the Business Case for Change

The design group soon realized that two issues would need to be addressed before a meaningful change in the profile of activities could begin to occur: (1) administrative support and (2) span of control. Years ago in a cost-cutting move, Metropolitan had eliminated nearly all unit secretaries, reasoning that they weren't really necessary any longer because nursing staff could enter patient information into the computer system themselves. Since then, management staff had had no administrative support.

Once the percentage of managerial time had been objectively determined, it was possible to price out the cost of getting those administrative tasks done. The design group was able to make a solid business case for using that 20 percent of each patient care manager's time to fund more administrative support. Even if the time freed up only resulted in a 1 percent savings in the cost of turnover, the results would more than pay for themselves. Finally, in addressing the issue of span of control, the design group ultimately convinced administration to commit $2.5 million over the next three years to increase the number of patient care managers. Given the fact that Metropolitan was spending $8.5 million per year on travelers to fill nursing vacancies, the design group was able to make the case that reductions in turnover would fund the increased overhead. Administration's leap of faith was rewarded: Eighteen months into the effort, use of travelers had been reduced by 33 percent, for an annualized savings of $2.8 million.

Typically, it requires a commitment of additional resources to address the kinds of issues that have made healthcare an increasingly unattractive industry in which to work. Teams that take on the challenge of reversing the tide will need to learn to build a business case for change. They'll also need access to trends and current information on expenditures for recruiting, agency staff, and overtime to spotlight costs built into the current scenario. Along these lines, the U.S. Department of Labor has estimated that the cost of turnover typically adds 33 percent to the fully loaded salary paid to a new hire. Assuming a 20 percent turnover rate, a conservative estimate for the cost of this turnover is $375,000 for every 100 nurses on staff annually. And that doesn't include the indirect costs—the hiring incentives, lost productivity, and the negative impact on patient and physician satisfaction. From this perspective, most hospitals cannot afford the status quo.

In addition to the need for a financially based business case, another useful tactic to build into plans for change is to structure resource commitments so that they can be self-funding. Carve out a pilot program and track metrics carefully. The savings realized can become a claim on continuing funding as well as a compelling argument for more.

Over the course of its first 18 months, the committee focused heavily on the patient care manager role. The dramatic disparity between the "as is" and "to be" role prompted the committee to develop a detailed action plan for changing the conditions that perpetuated the status quo. With new resource commitments that enabled reductions in the span of control and increase in administrative support, the committee created a task group that worked with human resources to ensure that the managers that they hired would be both capable and interested in implementing the patient care manager role in the way that the committee redefined it.

Leveraging Role Clarity to Enhance Procurement and Development

The task group worked with external consulting support to develop a competency profile from the patient care manager job charter. In the competency profile, each key accountability in the job charter had a corresponding section that showed the specific behavioral tasks a candidate needed to be able to do to deliver on that key accountability. Human resources then reworked this profile into a behaviorally based interview guide that would help interviewers drill down into a candidate's experience to assess whether the candidate had that particular competency. The expectation was that a better selection process, even when used to evaluate internal candidates, would yield more effective patient care managers who would want to stay in their jobs.

The task group also used the competency profile as a basis for creating a competency review process for current patient care managers. For the process, each patient care manager rated his or her level of effectiveness in each of the competencies in the profile. Their manager did the same, then both parties discussed their respective ratings to arrive at a consensus. The end result was a behaviorally based list of tasks that each current patient care manager needed to become more effective in their role. As important was that the process forced a dialog about current effectiveness, developmental needs, and career development.

Once the first such round of discussions had been completed, analysis of the consensus scores for all the patient care managers pointed at those tasks that were highest priority for the group as a whole. The group worked with training to develop programs that were responsive to these specific needs.

Systemic Change Requires Focus, Discipline, and Follow-Through

It's important to realize that effecting a systemic turnaround is a complex job. The team that spearheads the effort cannot possibly do everything that needs to be done on its own. Team members will be needed on an ad hoc basis or even on other specialty task teams for their expertise, so senior management support and sponsorship is critical. The job of those driving the larger effort is to prioritize and structure the tasks and deliverables in such circumstances, to hold people accountable for completing their assignments, to maintain focus on the larger goal, and to not allow themselves or those whose assistance they need to be distracted by day-to-day crises.

As the committee at Metropolitan Healthcare pursued the factors that helped to maintain the status quo for patient care managers, one of the issues that kept coming up was the volume of meetings that managers were expected to attend. Data from the activity study had indicated that patient care managers spent an average of 22 percent of their time attending meetings outside their units. Meetings with unit staff, in contrast, occupied less than 1 percent of their time. A quick survey identified 87 committees, many of which were standing, that had staff representation across the hospital. Aside from the sheer number and inclusiveness of committees, a review of those committees that kept minutes (which were few) and interview data clearly indicated that most did not function very effectively. It was clear that a major obstacle to patient care managers' reallocation of their time was cultural.

The committee took on the task of changing expectations and accepted practices regarding meeting management. Each committee in the hospital was required to draft a charter and a set of 12-month objectives. A committee management task force reviewed these charters and objectives; interviewed each committee head; and recommended whether continuation of the committee was warranted and, if so, whether changes in structure, meeting frequency, or membership should be made. In addition, the task force developed a set of policies on committee management that specified standard procedures that all remaining committees were required to follow, such as distributing agendas, taking minutes, and giving periodic plan and status updates. In conjunction with training, a meeting management workshop was developed that all committee heads and all patient care managers were required to attend.

As a result of the review, the number of committees was reduced from 87 to 36. When an activity study was repeated two years into the effort, results indicated that the time patient care managers spent on external committee activity had been cut nearly in half, down to 12 percent. Some of the recaptured time had gone into internal unit meetings. Employee survey data showed significant increases in the perceived quality of internal communication and coordination within the unit, in the level of process improvement that took place within the unit, and in the responsiveness of unit management to concerns of staff.

Follow the Data to Results

The course of activity to improve the quality of the work environment will vary from hospital to hospital. There is no standard order in which the six pillars discussed earlier need to be addressed. Each situation calls for its own diagnosis, and the course of action will vary based on the situation. As in our example, the team spearheading the effort needs to be prepared to go where the data lead them. The answer is often not a single change but a combination of new expectations; new policies and accountability; and, often, training to ensure that people have the skills they are being asked to use.

Thirty months into the retention management effort, the committee could look back at a track record of meaningful change. They had extended the job chartering process to a total of seven key positions, including the clinical educator, clinical nurse specialist, clinical (shift) manager, administrative director, vice president, and off-shift administrator. The committee had identified and prioritized core processes and successfully redesigned and standardized several that were critical to patient safety and satisfaction, one of which was the pain management process. Patient satisfaction data had raised the flag on this issue. High levels of demand for pain medication had strained the ability of the staff to be responsive. The situation was exacerbated by the fact that there was no consistent protocol followed across units for assessing, managing, and reporting pain. A redesign team mapped the pain management process used across the various units, bringing in unit staff to help explain each and its unique elements. In the end, the redesign team developed a common process, with a standardized protocol for assessment and reporting, that could be used across the hospital. In the six months since, patient pain reports had dropped by 20 percent.

The committee had also tackled the medication administration and documentation process. The effort to optimize and standardize core practices dovetailed well with JCAHO's review, which found that the hospital's medication errors were up and its processes were highly variable. As a starting point, the redesign team identified those units with higher numbers of incident reports and analyzed the underlying causes. With that as context, the team reviewed the process and its local variants and was able to develop a streamlined process that took less time, even though it incorporated additional check points. The team rolled out a training session to ensure that all staff understood the new process and added a module on measurement and dosing calculation, which the team's research had shown to be a contributing problem. Finally, the team raised the profile of the process by tracking incident reports weekly, working through patient care managers to ensure that policies were in fact followed. The results were gratifying: incident reports dropped by 50 percent.

Over the course of those 30 months, an environmental task force had established new standards across the hospital for cleaning patient rooms and public areas. A model room was developed, and orientation of new environmental assistants was revamped to include the use of the model room as a teaching tool. Environmental assistants no longer "floated" but were mapped to specific areas of the hospital, attended staff meetings on the units, and were given feedback based on an audit system developed with their input and implemented by patient care managers. The new audit system provided a total score on each room cleaned, a cumulative score for each month, and counts by checklist item to highlight tasks that were consistently substandard.

The biggest payoff for the committee was the improvement in retention. In nursing, position vacancies had dropped from 16 percent to 7 percent. The use of agency personnel dropped off accordingly, netting budgetary savings approaching $4 million annually, compared to expenditures before the project began. Turnover for the hospital had dropped from 24 percent to 14 percent, and even acceptance rates on job offers had increased. Employee survey data showed consistent improvements in employee identification with Metropolitan Healthcare and higher satisfaction with the environment and with management. Detailed questions on the behavior of managers clearly indicated that more constructive interaction was taking place and that employees were responding positively.

Most of the staff had grown to accept and even welcome the changes that had been made, although for some the new structure had been a hard adjustment because they were accustomed to defining their roles in ways that they personally found most comfortable. For some, the new structure precipitated their departure, either at their own initiative or by invitation. Once it became clear that administration was determined to make the new structure work, staff increasingly embraced the idea of change.

Setting Realistic Expectations

Systemic turnarounds take time. A realistic time frame for substantial improvement is 36 months. Even then, consider that time frame the first round. Because of the broad range of tactical objectives involved and the long time frames, retention management efforts put a premium on the ability of project team members to create and maintain structure. Effective project planning and management is a key requirement for progress against such large objectives. The team must reach agreement on what the barriers are to closing the gap between the current and desired future role; develop a clear picture of what needs to be accomplished to close the gap; and then break out tasks, time frames, and ownership of each step along the way. Regular meetings to review progress against plan and to solve obstacles are necessary for success. Finally, the ability to use influence effectively at the one-on-one level and through communication with various constituencies is a critical component of successful implementation.

Expectations for such a change effort must be carefully managed. What needs to be done will always exceed the resources available, so the project team needs to constantly prioritize and keep administration informed. Because retention is a function of so many elements, the critical path to success is not always clear. It helps to realize that retention management is an iterative process and as long as the project team can learn from its successes, and failures, the outcome will inevitably be a positive one for the hospital and its workforce.

CONCLUSION

This chapter analyzes the complex factors that have brought us to our current state of affairs and, perhaps more importantly, provides a roadmap for finding our way back. The six pillars that support patient care effectiveness offer guidance to administrators and project managers on how to "map" the current situation into manageable, coherent segments and how to prioritize addressing each one. The chapter also illustrates, through a composite but realistic case example, the type and sequence of diagnostic and remedial steps that will most likely be useful to any hospital with retention problems today. In addition, it offers guidance for incorporating principles of change management and for managing expectations of various publics in connection with such an undertaking.

Epilog

The sources of our current problems in healthcare are many and varied—an interweaving of "baby boom" demographics; societal change opening new doors to women; economic pressures to contain spiraling healthcare costs; and well-intentioned, if not always effective, efforts to apply lessons learned from production environments to the healthcare business.

The path to making our healthcare industry a more attractive environment in which to work is likewise complex. Just as the current situation derives from a systemic interaction of factors, so will the solution. Going well beyond narrowly focused attempts to address employee concerns in isolation, the key to improved retention of staff in our hospitals will be to address the range of needs that all employees have for structure, stability, predictability, and challenges that they can successfully manage and feel good about. While buy-in and participation have their place in the solution, they are not by themselves the answer. In most hospitals today, fundamental assumptions will need to be challenged and changed, on the part of both employees and administrators, before the exodus of employees will moderate. What will be required is greater focus, discipline, and follow through than has typically characterized management in healthcare, with thoughtful adherence to the principles of change management to realign expectations and outcomes. We are hopeful that the industry is ready to embrace some longer-term solutions before our position as the world's preeminent healthcare system is seriously eroded.

The Six Pillars

1. Ensure role clarity through job charters and competencies that define expectations of individuals' roles and their role on a multidisciplinary team.
2. Establish optimal structures, focus on clear accountability for excellence, and provide support for development to achieve goals.
3. Establish excellent core processes and standardize practices that cut across all services to increase efficiency, increase effectiveness, and lower costs, building in custom processes where needed.
4. Ensure real-time availability of appropriate equipment, supplies, and tools to deliver excellence.
5. Create a patient-centered environment where safety, cleanliness, customer service, and excellence in patient outcomes are expected and delivered reliably.
6. Design multiple patient care delivery models that meet the needs of distinctly different patient populations.

About the Authors

Rita E. Numerof, Ph.D., is president of Numerof & Associates, Inc. (NAI), a strategic management consulting firm based in St. Louis, Missouri. An internationally recognized consultant and author, Dr. Numerof brings over 20 years of experience in the field of strategy execution, process excellence, and organizational development to her work as author and advisor to major corporations.

Dr. Numerof's career has included experience as a hospital administrator, clinician, academician, and director of a healthcare MBA program. Through NAI, her work spans a wide variety of industries, including financial services, manufacturing, and utilities, but healthcare remains a major focus.

Dr. Numerof works with *Fortune* 500 clients across a variety of industries and healthcare organizations to implement systemic and operational change in support of strategy execution. Her experience ranges from operations and process infrastructure design and development to market strategy, planning, and integration. Her coaching and management/executive development activities address the challenges of creating linkage to strategic objectives, accountability for results, and the creation of work environments that support innovation and quality. She has facilitated Six Sigma initiatives that led to breakthrough improvements in performance, designed executive development programs, and guided organizations in the design and implementation of cultural change strategies that increase operational effectiveness and employee retention.

Dr. Numerof is an entertaining and provocative speaker and a widely published management author and commentator. She has authored four books and serves as an adjunct faculty member for the Olin School of Business at Washington University in St. Louis. Dr. Numerof graduated magna cum laude from the Honors College at Syracuse University and received her M.S.S. and Ph.D. degrees from Bryn Mawr College. She is listed in Who's Who of American Women and Who's Who Among Top Executives.

Michael N. Abrams, M.A., is vice president and managing partner of Numerof & Associates, Inc. (NAI). He has served as an internal and external consultant to *Fortune* 500 corporations, major financial and service organizations, healthcare institutions, and state and federal government agencies for more than 20 years. He has worked extensively in the areas of operational assessment, market analysis, strategic planning, human resource systems design, and management and organizational development. By addressing issues of planning, process management, structure and measurement, Mr. Abrams has assisted clients in the healthcare field in balancing the interests of patients, physicians, and employees with the need for financial viability. His publications and consulting experience are noted for their focus on organizational assessment and change in the context of strategic business planning.

Mr. Abrams is well known for his expertise in the design and implementation of systems and surveys for managing productivity, assessing and managing organizational climate, and assessing and managing customer needs and expectations. His ability to identify market opportunities and effectively address service gaps has been an invaluable resource to client companies. Most significantly he has been successful in structuring and managing the internal change processes necessary to translate business opportunities into effective operations and new product design.

Mr. Abrams is a widely published author in management journals and a frequent presenter to business audiences throughout the country. As an adjunct faculty member, Mr. Abrams has taught MBA courses in management and marketing, program planning and evaluation, and quantitative decision making. Mr. Abrams completed his doctoral course work in policy analysis at St. Louis University. He received his M.A. from George Washington University in Washington, D.C.